LWW'S PHARMACY TECHNICIAN
Certification Exam Review

Sandra Tschritter, B.A., C.Ph.T.

Spokane Community College

⊕ Wolters Kluwer | Lippincott Williams & Wilkins
Health

Philadelphia • Baltimore • New York • London
Buenos Aires • Hong Kong • Sydney • Tokyo

Acquisitions Editor: David B. Troy
Product Manager: Renee Thomas
Marketing Manager: Allison Powell
Designer: Doug Smock
Compositor: Macmillan
Printer: RR Donnelley, China

First Edition

Library of Congress Cataloging-in-Publication Data
Tschritter, Sandra.
  LWW's pharmacy technician certification exam review / Sandra Tschritter.—1st ed.
      p. ; cm.
   Other title: Pharmacy technician certification exam review
   Includes bibliographical references and index.
   ISBN 978-0-7817-9633-0 (alk. paper)
   1. Pharmacy technicians—Examinations, questions, etc. 2. Pharmacy technicians—Outlines, syllabi, etc. I. Title. II. Title: Pharmacy technician certification exam review.
   [DNLM: 1. Pharmacy—Examination Questions. 2. Pharmaceutical Services—Examination Questions. 3. Pharmacists' Aides. QV 18.2 T879L 2011]
   RS122.95.T73 2011
   615'.1076—dc22   2010011425

DISCLAIMER

Care has been taken to confirm the accuracy of the information present and to describe generally accepted practices. However, the authors, editors, and publisher are not responsible for errors or omissions or for any consequences from application of the information in this book and make no warranty, expressed or implied, with respect to the currency, completeness, or accuracy of the contents of the publication. Application of this information in a particular situation remains the professional responsibility of the practitioner; the clinical treatments described and recommended may not be considered absolute and universal recommendations.

The authors, editors, and publisher have exerted every effort to ensure that drug selection and dosage set forth in this text are in accordance with the current recommendations and practice at the time of publication. However, in view of ongoing research, changes in government regulations, and the constant flow of information relating to drug therapy and drug reactions, the reader is urged to check the package insert for each drug for any change in indications and dosage and for added warnings and precautions. This is particularly important when the recommended agent is a new or infrequently employed drug.

Some drugs and medical devices presented in this publication have Food and Drug Administration (FDA) clearance for limited use in restricted research settings. It is the responsibility of the health care provider to ascertain the FDA status of each drug or device planned for use in their clinical practice.

To purchase additional copies of this book, call our customer service department at (800) 638-3030 or fax orders to (301) 223-2320. International customers should call (301) 223-2300.
Visit Lippincott Williams & Wilkins on the Internet: http://www.lww.com. Lippincott Williams & Wilkins customer service representatives are available from 8:30 am to 6:00 pm, EST.

Preface

LWW's Pharmacy Technician Certification Exam Review is designed to help students and technicians preparing to take the certification exam offered by the Pharmacy Technician Certification Board (PTCB) as well as other certification exams such as the Exam for the Certification of Pharmacy Technicians (ExCPT), which is offered by the Institute for the Certification of Pharmacy Technicians. The content and questions in this text cover all the knowledge statements of the PTCB and all the key subject areas of the exams.

LWW's Pharmacy Technician Certification Exam Review is thoughtfully organized to be the best choice for students and technicians. The text is presented in three Parts according to the major duties of pharmacy technicians: Assisting the Pharmacist in Serving Patients, Maintaining Medication and Inventory Control Systems, and Participating in the Administration and Management of Pharmacy Practice.

The content is divided into 16 chapters covering the subject areas of the exams. Each chapter includes the following features:

- **Test Topics** clearly state the exam topics included in the chapter, setting the stage for productive studying.

- **Test Terms** are valuable study tools for students and technicians that are listed and defined at the beginning of the chapter, boldfaced in the text at first use, and included in the glossary at the end of the text.

- **Exam content coverage** in each chapter uses a "quick review" approach to give the reader a chance to brush up on key concepts before moving on to the practice questions.

- **Practice Test Questions** are the bulk of each chapter, made up of multiple-choice questions to help the reader practice taking exam-like questions.

- **Recall Tips** provide reminders and mnemonic devices for the reader to help remember specific facts.

Other important advantages of *LWW's Pharmacy Technician Certification Exam Review* are:

- **A whole chapter devoted to exam preparation and study tips.** The first chapter in the book offers tips on how to study and prepare for the exam as well as strategies to keep in mind while taking the exam.

- **A whole chapter devoted to math.** Many students and technicians find math the most difficult aspect of the exam as well as practice. This text provides concise, focused review and extra practice questions.

- **A complete practice exam included in the text.** In addition to the practice questions in each chapter, students can prepare by taking a 125-question multiple choice exam.

- **Electronic Quiz Bank available on bound-in CD-ROM as well as on *thePoint* website.*** With 600 questions, the Quiz Bank includes Review Mode for instant feedback and Exam Mode for exam-like conditions.

*See the inside front cover of this text for more details, including the passcode you will need to gain access to the website: http://thePoint.lww.com/Tschritter.

Reviewers

The authors and publisher wish to thank the following people for their invaluable feedback on this text.

Mary Arnold

Wytheville Community College
Wytheville, VA

Julette Barta

Colton-Redland-Yucaipa Regional Occupational Program
Redlands, CA

Christy Bivins

North Georgia Technical College
Clarkesville, GA

Thomas Fridley

Sanford Brown Institute
New York, NY

Janet McGregor Liles

Arkansas State University-Beebe
Beebe, AR

Traci Tonhofer

Davis Applied Technology College
Kaysville, UT

Richard Witt

Alleghany College of Maryland
Cumberland, MD

Contents

Reviewers iii

Preface v

CHAPTER 1 / Preparing for the Exam 1

Part I / Assisting the Pharmacist in Serving Patients 11

CHAPTER 2 / Law and Ethics 12

CHAPTER 3 / Medical Abbreviations and Terminology 22

CHAPTER 4 / Anatomy, Physiology, and Disease 33

CHAPTER 5 / Pharmacology 42

CHAPTER 6 / Dosage Forms, Delivery Systems, and Routes of Administration 50

CHAPTER 7 / Pharmacy Calculations and Measurement Systems 58

CHAPTER 8 / Sterile Products and Pharmacy Equipment 71

CHAPTER 9 / Preparation of Non-Sterile products 82

CHAPTER 10 / Dispensing Medications 90

Part II / Maintaining Medication and Inventory Control Systems 97

CHAPTER 11 / Inventory Management and Handling and Storage of Medications 98

Part III / Participating in the Administration and Management of Pharmacy Practice 107

CHAPTER 12 / Administrative Duties and Technology 108

CHAPTER 13 / Business Management 120

CHAPTER 14 / Professionalism and Personnel Management 132

CHAPTER 15 / Infection Control and Hazardous Materials 143

CHAPTER 16 / Facility Management 157

Appendix A: Answers to Chapter Practice Test Questions 169

Appendix B: Practice Exam 191

Appendix C: Practice Exam Answer Key 198

Glossary 199

1

Preparing for the Exam

Test Topics

After completing this chapter, you should be able to demonstrate knowledge of the following:

1. Purpose of the Pharmacy Technician Certification Board
2. Background information on the Pharmacy Technician Certification Exam
3. Various strategies to implement when studying for the certification exam
4. Tips and techniques to use when taking a multiple-choice exam

Test Terms

- **Certified Pharmacy Technicians (CPhT)** credential given to pharmacy technicians who have passed the Pharmacy Technician Certification Exam (PTCE); initial certification and recertification last for two years
- **Pharmacy Technician Certification Board (PTCB)** governing body that was formed in 1995 to establish national standards for pharmacy technician certification
- **Pharmacy Technician Certification Exam (PTCE)** certification exam designed to test the skills required for pharmacy technicians; after passing the exam, a pharmacy technician is certified by the Pharmacy Technician Certification Board (PTCB)

A pharmacy technician's primary purpose is to assist the pharmacist in tasks that do not require a fully trained pharmacist's judgment and discretion. Not all states require certification for pharmacy technicians; however it is strongly recommended for several reasons.

- Studying for and passing the certification exam will increase your knowledge of proper pharmacy practices and your ability to best assist the pharmacist.
- Your knowledge of proper practices will decrease the likelihood of making a medication error that could compromise the health of a client.
- Most pharmacies in retail stores and hospitals are more likely to hire a certified technician, particularly when hiring someone who does not have prior pharmacy experience.

In this chapter, you will learn about the Pharmacy Technician Certification Board, which oversees the certification process for pharmacy technicians. The ultimate goal of this book is to provide you with the skills and knowledge needed to pass the certification examination, and this chapter will also cover helpful studying and test-taking strategies.

The Pharmacy Technician Certification Board

The body that develops the exam and controls the certification process is the **Pharmacy Technician Certification Board (PTCB)**. The PTCB was formed in January 1995 to establish a national standard for pharmacy technician certification. It is governed by five organizations:

- The American Pharmacists Association
- The American Society of Health System Pharmacists
- The Illinois Council of Health System Pharmacists
- The Michigan Pharmacists Association
- The National Association of Boards of Pharmacy

There was no nationally standardized certification process for pharmacy technicians before the PTCB was developed. Now there is a certification process that is recognized by the profession in most states (some states do not required standardized education or testing). This approach is consistent with the pharmacist licensure process, and makes it easier to establish guidelines for the accreditation of schools that offer pharmacy technician certification courses.

Summary of Mission and Vision Statements

The official mission of the PTCB is to develop, maintain, promote, and administer a high quality certification and recertification program for pharmacy technicians. The vision of the board is to support a set of credentials in the practice setting that are the same nationwide. The skills and knowledge developed from studying for and passing the certification exam will help pharmacy technicians to work effectively with pharmacists. Strong teamwork between pharmacists and technicians is essential in providing the best possible pharmaceutical care for patients. The PTCB feels that Certified Pharmacy Technicians (CPhTs) are the best support for pharmacists in ensuring safe, accurate, and efficient medication distribution. The PTCB hopes to produce the best possible pharmacy technicians by developing and maintaining a high quality, practice-based certification examination.

The Certification Exam

You must sit for and pass the **Pharmacy Technician Certification Exam (PTCE)** in order to receive PTCB certification. After passing the exam, you can use the title **Certified Pharmacy Technician (CPhT)**. The certification is valid for two years, during which time a CPhT must obtain twenty hours of continuing education, of which at least one must be in pharmacy law, in order to be recertified. Recertification is also valid for two years. It is important to maintain certification, as most hospitals and retail pharmacy chains require it to continue working there.

In order to be eligible for the exam, applicants must have a high school diploma or its equivalent. In addition, the PTCB's other requirements for eligibility are that applicants have not been convicted of a felony within the last five years; have not had their license suspended, revoked, or restricted by the State Board of Pharmacy; and have not been convicted of any drug- or pharmacy-related crimes.

The exam is designed to test the skills that an actual pharmacy technician would use on a daily basis in the pharmacy. Content for the exam was drawn from a nationwide study of the work that pharmacy technicians perform. The study was based on a variety of practice settings, including community and institutional pharmacies. Hospital pharmacy work can be somewhat more difficult than retail, as orders for medication need to be filled immediately in emergency situations, and the volume of orders can be much greater in a busy hospital. Getting a job at a hospital pharmacy almost always requires current certification and prior experience.

Components of the Exam

There are 100 multiple-choice questions on the exam, ten of which are "pre-test" questions. These ten questions are scattered throughout the test at random, and are used to provide statistical information for possible use on future exams. They may or may not be part of a future version of the pharmacy technician certification exam, depending on the difficulty level of and student success rate on these questions. The goal of the test is not to trick you into picking the wrong answer, but rather to ensure that you have the knowledge necessary to be a competent assistant for a pharmacist. In order to pass, you must receive a score of at least 650 on the exam.

Exam questions are designed to cover three basic areas:

- assisting the pharmacist in serving patients (66% of the exam)
- maintaining medication and inventory control systems (22% of the exam)
- participating in the administration and management of pharmacy practice (12% of the exam)

These three content areas cover the basic functions of a pharmacy technician, and mastery of these will ensure that you will be a competent technician.

Practice Exams

There is a practice exam included in Appendix B of this book, as well as additional practice exams on the CD-ROM accompanying this book and on the book's companion website (thePoint.lww.com/Tschritter). The PTCB Web site (www.ptcb.org) offers a practice exam to familiarize you with the format and possible content of the official exam you will take.

Taking the practice exams and studying the answers to them is a useful tool in preparing yourself for the actual exam. Although the content on the actual exam will vary, the material is essentially the same, and being familiar with the practice exams will certainly be an advantage at test time. The PTCB Web site also has additional information about the test, the board, and the answers to general questions that you may have about the responsibilities and requirements of being a pharmacy technician.

Registering for the Exam

As of the date of this publication, the registration fee for the PTCB exam is $129. This is refundable if you must cancel, as long as you do so at least 24 hours prior to the scheduled exam date. Students are given two hours to complete the exam, which consists of 100 multiple choice questions. This allows you one minute and twenty seconds to answer each question. In the past, the exam was offered once per every 6 to 8 week period throughout the year. In April of 2009, the PTCB began offering continuous testing cycles, so the exam is available every day. You can register for the exam on the PTCB Web site, and information about testing centers and times that are most convenient for you is also available on the site.

Taking the Exam

There are several different versions of the test given at the same time, in an effort to avoid cheating. While the questions are not identical, they cover the same basic subject matter. No one version of the test is intended to be more difficult than another. The exam is computerized in a simple format that does not require the test-taker to have extensive computer skills. Every testing center gives a brief tutorial before the test is administered about how to properly take the computerized exam. Remember, you will not be allowed to bring aids such as scrap paper or calculators in to the test. After taking the test, you will receive a printout that tells you the date when your scores and your "pass/fail" status will be available. If you fail the exam the first time, you must wait 90 days before taking it again.

Recertification

Recertification, as mentioned before, is required every two years. In order to maintain certification you must complete twenty hours of continuing education within the two-year certification period. At least one hour of this must cover pharmacy law. The PTCB does not offer official continuing education courses, but does provide a list of approved continuing education providers on its Web site. You can use one college course per two-year period as part of your continuing education. The course must be in a Life Science (Chemistry, Biology, Anatomy, etc.) or Math. A college course will count for fifteen of your twenty continuing education hours for that time period. Continuing education is also available online via web seminars such as www.DrugTopics.com or www.pharmacychoice.com, or through pharmacy journals such as *Technician Today*, which is published by NPTA journal of Pharmacy Technology.

Remember, Continuing education must be completed before the two-year certification period is up. There is a 90-day grace period to submit continuing education paperwork after certification has expired. If the paperwork is not submitted within that period of time, an applicant has to complete a full reinstatement process, the details of which are available on the PTCB Web site.

Alternative to PCTB Exam

In addition to the PCTB Exam, another accepted certification exam is known as the ExCPT, or the Exam for the Certification of Pharmacy Technicians. The exam is administered by the Institute for the Certificate of Pharmacy Technicians (ICPT), an accredited organization recognized by the NCPA (National Community Pharmacy Association). Similar to the PCTE, recertification under ExCPT must be completed every two years. The technician must also complete at least 20 hours of continuing education during that time.

Honing Your Study Skills

The concept of studying is simple: reread your books and notes and commit the important concepts to memory. But what does it really mean to study, and how does one study effectively? Studying is:

- refreshing your memory
- taking in new information
- organizing and memorizing data

When studying for a large, comprehensive examination like the PTCE, there is a lot of new information to be taken in, organized, and recalled for the test, and hopefully retained so you can use it on the job. It's no surprise that many students sit down to study and find themselves feeling overwhelmed. Any little distraction can keep you from studying effectively and efficiently. That's why it's important to study the right way.

Find an Appropriate Study Area

The first thing you need to do is find a good place to study. Look for a location that is free of distractions. Also, make sure the area is large enough for you to arrange all your study materials. Think about any furniture you might need, such as a desk or large table.

Some students prefer to sit at a table when they study. This arrangement keeps them alert and focused, while helping them keep their materials organized. They can put the study materials they're using on the table and keep materials they'll need later underneath it. Other students might feel more comfortable sitting on a sofa, with their study materials on a coffee table or spread out on the floor below. One place you may want to avoid studying, if possible, is your bedroom. If you're tired, your bed may be too tempting to resist.

After you've come up with several possible study areas, compare each space in terms of the lighting, temperature, and other surroundings. Think about two or three areas that might make good study spaces. Then choose the one place that has the most favorable responses to these questions.

- Are there a lot of other people in the same space who could interrupt me?
- Are there things in the space that will distract me from studying?
- Is there a TV or radio in the space that might be turned on?
- Is there a phone that might ring too often?
- Is this space easy for me to get to on a regular basis?
- Is the temperature comfortable? If it isn't, can I change it?
- Is this space big enough so it won't get cluttered when I spread out all my materials?
- Is there enough light so I can read without straining my eyes?

Prepare Your Mind and Body

Once you have found the most appropriate study area, it is time to prepare your mind and body to study. Your brain is part of your body. If your body is uncomfortable, your brain has a harder time properly focusing. When you're studying, you need your brain to focus fully on your work, not your aching back. You can stay comfortable by having good posture, avoiding eyestrain, moving around, and eating healthy snacks during long study sessions. Here are some ways to stay alert and be comfortable as you study.

- Sit up straight to keep your back and neck from getting stiff. It's worth the effort, and it can become a habit if you stick with it. Sitting up straight also keeps you alert and helps you concentrate.
- Make sure your reading material is propped up at about a 45-degree angle from your work surface. And keep your eyes at least 15 inches away from what you're reading. If you're too close, your eyes can't focus properly. If you're too far away, you'll strain forward.
- Don't forget to get up and walk around every so often when you're studying. Stay in your study area, but try pacing around, doing jumping jacks, or performing simple stretching exercises. When you stand, 5 to 15 percent more blood flows to your brain. This means your brain gets more oxygen and stays stimulated.
- Nutrition is essential for optimal brain function. If you're going to study for more than an hour at a time, bring a healthy and easy snack, like grapes, so you can eat without mess or distraction.

Improve Your Concentration

We've already talked a little about the distractions that can interfere with your study time. There are external distractions, like noises, which can cause you to lose your concentration. There are internal distractions as well, like hunger or anxiety, which can make studying difficult.

You can learn to improve your concentration skills so you can overcome those distractions. But it takes motivation to improve your concentration. You must want to learn the material in front of you. It might help to remember why it is important for your future career. Your desire to learn will help you stay focused on studying. Also, you need to be awake, alert, and prepared to learn. Being alert the first time you study helps you avoid multiple unnecessary review sessions.

Improving your concentration during study time also helps you remember more material. This means you will increase your chances of passing the PTCE. Here are some tips that will help you concentrate and study effectively:

- Take a short walk, about five to ten minutes long, to clear your head and relax your body.
- Meditate for about five minutes. Sit quietly, perhaps in your study area with the lights off. Sit up straight and picture something still and peaceful. Breathe deeply and slowly.
- Try to avoid caffeine. Too much can cause you to become jumpy and make it harder to concentrate.
- Study during a time of day when you're awake and alert.
- Focus on one topic at a time.
- Keep your brain active by engaging in different activities, such as reading, taking notes, and spending time thinking.
- Take short breaks every 45 minutes to one hour.

As with so many things, practice makes perfect when it comes to concentration. It might seem discouraging if you get distracted easily the first few times you attempt to study. If you keep at it, however, you'll train your brain to stay focused.

Improve Your Memory Skills

Information is stored in different ways in your brain. That's why it's easy to remember some events or people and harder to remember others. Memory isn't a sense; it's a skill you can develop and improve. By understanding how memory works, you can learn ways to improve it. The three stages of information processing are:

1. *Registration.* During this stage the brain receives information, recognizes what you have experienced and gives it meaning, and chooses which pieces of the information to remember.
2. *Short-term memory.* After information is processed by your brain, it moves into short-term memory. However, short-term memory cannot hold a great deal of information, and what it can hold doesn't stay for long. By grouping important information, you can make space for more data in your short-term memory.
3. *Long-term memory.* After information is grouped, your brain either forgets it or moves it to long-term memory, where it is organized and stored for long periods of time.

The term *working memory* describes how your brain stores and retrieves information from short-term and long-term memory. Improving your working memory is critical to remembering what you study. You can use four strategies to improve your working memory. These are:

- *Selection.* Selection consists of singling out the most important information that you need to remember.
- *Association.* Association means linking a new piece of information to something you already know. For example, if you are trying to remember that a certain patient is allergic to a medication, you may remember your mother's allergy to cats when thinking of this patient.
- *Organization.* Organization involves breaking new information into groups that will help your brain store the information. Remembering a string of seven numbers

(such as 1-9-4-6-3-2-0) can be difficult, but if you break the numbers into two groups (such as 1946 and 320), it becomes much easier.

- *Rehearsal.* The last strategy is rehearsal, which is simply repeatedly reviewing the information that you have learned.

Use Study Strategies

There are many study strategies that can help you recall information later during tests. You've already read about a few of these strategies. Using a variety of study methods helps your brain take in and store the same information in different ways. This creates multiple pathways for your brain to use when you're trying to recall the information later. Below are some recommended study strategies.

- *Practice.* Repeat information out loud, write the same material several times, or read and then reread information silently.
- *Take breaks.* Intermittent breaks give you immediate rewards for hard work, help you complete manageable amounts of work, and keep information moving from working memory to long-term memory.
- *Use acronyms and acrostics.* An acronym is a word created from using the first letter of each item on a list. Acrostics are phrases in which the first letter of each word stands for something else. Pharmacy technicians could use the acrostic "Old Dogs Rest" to remember the three times to check a medicine you are preparing. ("o" represents taking the drug out of the container, "d" represents placing medication in the dispenser, and "r" represents returning the drug to storage.)
- *Reduce interference.* Study in a peaceful location.
- *Create lists.* Lists help you organize information.
- *Use imagery.* Try to imagine a mental picture of the information you are learning.
- *Create flash cards.* Break the information down into basic ideas that you can study in short bursts or on-the-go.

Rest, Relax, and Eat Right

As you study, your brain needs time to sort information and store it in your memory. To do that, your brain needs rest. During deep sleep, the brain keeps right on sorting and storing information, saving important information and forgetting unimportant details. By getting enough rest and relaxation, your brain can take a break from processing information, allowing it to catch up. Eating a healthy, balanced diet is also essential in maintaining optimal brain function.

Test-Taking Tips

Your score on the PTCE is the single deciding factor in whether or not you receive pharmacy technician certification. Tests with this kind of real-life significance attached to them can cause students a lot of anxiety. In this section, you will learn how to plan and prepare for the exam so you can improve your test-taking abilities and feel more confident. You will also learn some skills to help manage excessive test anxiety.

Recognizing and Managing Test Anxiety

Are you an overly anxious test taker? There are many forms of test anxiety that come before and during a test. Here are some types of test anxiety:

- freezing up, when your brain doesn't take in the meaning of questions or you have to read questions repeatedly to understand them
- panicking about tough questions or about time running out before you're done

- worrying about the score you'll receive
- becoming easily distracted or daydreaming
- feeling nervous about your ability to do well or about how you'll do compared to others
- having physical symptoms of stress, such as sweating, nausea, muscle tension, and headaches

The key to staying on top of anxiety is using a combination of techniques to prepare for tests. This section discusses tips and tricks all students can use. It's also important to remember that you need to prepare your mind and body. Keeping this balance will help you overcome your test anxiety and do your best. Here are some strategies that will help you manage your test anxiety:

- Study well. Being thoroughly prepared for the exam is the best measure to overcome anxiety.
- Relax your mind. Try using breathing exercises or meditation to clear your mind.
- Think positively. Low self-esteem can cause anxiety; tell yourself that you will succeed.
- Give yourself a break. If you feel overwhelmed during the exam, consider doing something to break the tension, such as closing your eyes and taking a few deep breaths.
- Get enough sleep. Being well-rested is extremely important in avoiding anxiety.
- Sit up straight. Good posture reduces stress.
- Stay on schedule. Maintain your normal routine leading up to the exam.

Know What Will Be Covered on the Test

To learn more about the exam before you take it, attend class regularly, and ask your instructor questions about the exam. The practice exams included at the end of this book and on the PTCB Web site are great tools for familiarizing yourself with the format and content of the exam.

Strategies for Exam Day

After you have studied and reviewed thoroughly, there are a few strategies that will help you perform your best on exam day.

- Eat small meals. Breakfast is the most important.
- Avoid caffeine. You don't want to be jittery.
- Exercise. A short exercise session before the exam will help you feel mentally and physically invigorated.
- Arrive on time. Make sure you wear a watch. Not only will this help you avoid being late or having to rush to be on time, but during the test you can track how much time is left. It's best to arrive a little early so you can be seated and ready by the time the test begins.
- Pay attention to the exam instructions. Listen carefully before you rush right to the questions.
- Budget test time efficiently. Think about how much time you have to finish the exam and the total number of questions to be answered. If you start to lag during the exam, don't stress. You can rebound by adjusting your schedule.

Strategies for Success on Objective Tests

There is only one right answer for each question on an objective test. The point is to test your recall of facts. The Pharmacy Technician Certification Exam is comprised entirely of multiple-choice questions. Here are some strategies to help you decipher multiple-choice questions:

- Read each question carefully. Phrases like *except*, *not*, and *all of the following* provide important clues to the correct answer.

- Try to answer each question before you look at the answer choices. Then, try to match your answer to one of the choices. Even if you feel you have a match at choice one, read the rest of the choices to see if there's an even closer match.

- Use the process of elimination to narrow your answer choices. Some answers are clearly wrong. Disregard those and focus on the ones that might be correct.

- Work quickly! You won't have time to answer truly hard questions if you take too long checking and double-checking the ones you think you answered correctly.

Chapter Summary

- The Pharmacy Technician Certification Board is the single national regulatory body that develops and maintains a certification process for Pharmacy Technicians.

- The goal of the PTCB is to establish a nationally standardized certification process for Pharmacy Technicians that tests applicants on knowledge and skills needed to be a competent technician.

- Applicants must not have committed a felony or pharmacy/drug related crime within the last five years to be eligible to sit for the exam.

- Certification is valid for two years, during which time pharmacy technicians must complete twenty hours of continuing education to be recertified.

- The exam has continuous registration, and the fee is $129. Testing centers are listed on the PTCB Web site, and offer a brief tutorial of how to take the computerized test prior to the exam.

- Test material is drawn from a national survey of the actual tasks performed by current pharmacy technicians.

- Study spaces should be comfortable, spacious, and free of distractions.

- Concentration can be improved with practice. Light exercise and meditation techniques can improve focus and concentration.

- Memory can be improved through methods like grouping information, association with things from your life, and the use of imagery.

- Proper rest and nutrition are essential in maintaining optimal brain function and effective studying.

- Effective preparation and studying are the best ways to combat test anxiety.

- When taking a multiple-choice test, don't spend too much time checking and double-checking the questions you think you answered correctly.

PART
1

Assisting the Pharmacist in Serving Patients

CHAPTER 2 / Law and Ethics

CHAPTER 3 / Medical Abbreviations and Terminology

CHAPTER 4 / Anatomy, Physiology, and Disease

CHAPTER 5 / Pharmacology

CHAPTER 6 / Dosage Forms, Delivery Systems, and Routes of Administration

CHAPTER 7 / Pharmacy Calculations and Measurement Systems

CHAPTER 8 / Sterile Products and Pharmacy Equipment

CHAPTER 9 / Preparation of Non-Sterile Products

CHAPTER 10 / Dispensing Medications

2

Law and Ethics

Test Topics

After completing this chapter, you should be able to demonstrate knowledge of the following:

1. Federal, state, and/or practice site regulations, codes of ethics, and standards pertaining to the practice of pharmacy
2. Pharmaceutical, medical, and legal developments that impact the practice of pharmacy
3. State-specific prescription transfer regulations
4. Confidentiality requirements

Test Terms

- **civil laws** laws that govern wrongdoings against a person or property, and generally charges are brought forth by another individual
- **Controlled Substances Act (CSA)** 1970 act that was designed to help regulate drug use by creating rules and regulations for record keeping and dispensing, and requiring firms that handled controlled substances to register with the DEA; the act also organized controlled substances into a system of schedules based on the potential for abuse
- **Drug Listing Act** 1972 act established to create a list of marketed drugs for the Food and Drug Administration, which would assist with enforcing federal safety laws
- **Durham-Humphrey Amendment (DHA)** 1951 amendment that separated drugs into two categories: legend drugs (prescriptions drugs) and over-the-counter drugs (OTC); the amendment specified that news drugs can only be distributed through prescriptions (and should contain legends to that effect), but eventually may be changed to OTC status
- **ethics** system of values, principles, and duties that guide behavior
- **Food, Drug, and Cosmetic Act (FDCA)** 1938 act that helped ensure drugs being distributed were safe and fulfilled the reported claim of strength, purity, and quality
- **Health Insurance Portability and Accountability Act (HIPAA)** act established in 1996 that requires healthcare providers to provide a clear written explanation of how health information will be used and disclosed
- **Kefauver-Harris Amendment (KHA)** 1962 amendment that became part of the Food, Drug, and Cosmetic Act; the amendment was designed to institute higher safety measures for drugs approved by the Food and Drug Administration by requiring manufacturers to follow Good Manufacturing Processes (GMP)
- **Orphan Drug Act** 1983 act created by the Food and Drug Administration to speed up the approval process for new medications intended to help people with urgent needs
- **Poison Prevention Packaging Act (PPPA)** 1970 act created to reduce potential for accidental poisonings

The study and practice of pharmacology covers many legal and ethical issues. Regulations regarding the practice of pharmacy can change, so it's important to keep track of new developments. Current laws being debated include the right to die and the legal use of marijuana. Visit your state's Board of Pharmacy Web site for development that may impact you.

Laws are rules regarding conduct that are enforced by an authority, such as the government. Pharmacology is generally regulated by civil laws. **Civil laws** govern wrongdoings against a person or property, and generally charges are brought forth by another individual.

Whereas laws are enforced by the government, ethics are enforced by peers, professional organizations, and the community. **Ethics** are a system of values, principles, and duties that guide your behavior. Your ethical commitments to your patients include:

- nonmalfeasance—actions that avoid harm
- beneficence—actions that create benefits
- fidelity—adherence to laws and agreements; meeting patients' rights to receive care and respect
- veracity—truth
- justice—equal allocation of burdens and benefits

Confidentiality

Confidentiality is not only an ethical issue; it's also ethical legal one. The **Health Insurance Portability and Accountability Act of 1996 (HIPAA)** was originally developed to make sure that people could not lose their medical coverage when they changed jobs, even if they had a pre-existing medical condition. Today, HIPAA affects almost all healthcare providers as well as anyone who is employed anywhere where patient information may be located, including pharmacies. Under HIPPA, the following information, which is also known as a patient's Protected Health Information (PHI) is considered confidential:

- names
- geographic location smaller than a state
- dates of birth, admission, discharge, or death
- telephone and fax numbers
- e-mail addresses
- Social Security numbers
- medical records or account numbers
- health plan beneficiary numbers
- certificate/license numbers
- vehicle or device numbers
- biometric indicators
- full face photos
- any other unique identifying number, characteristic, or code
- age older than 89

According to HIPAA, confidential information may only be released under one of the following circumstances:

- under written consent of the patient
- by subpoena
- in cases of mandatory reporting

RECALL TIP

Use the phrase "when to show medical records" to remember when confidential information can be released. "W" represents written consent of the patient, "s" represents subpoena, and "m" and "r" represent mandatory reporting.

Drug Regulations

A drug is defined as an agent intended for use in the diagnosis, mitigation, treatment, cure, or prevention of disease in humans or in other animals. The following sections describe drug regulations that have been implemented for public safety.

Food, Drug, and Cosmetic Act of 1938

RECALL TIP

To help remember what the Food, Drug, and Cosmetic Act is all about, remember the act's acronym, FDCA. "F" represents fulfilled, "d" represents description of, "c" represents claim, and "a" represents act. This way FDCA stands for Food, Drug, and Cosmetic Act, but it also stands for "fulfilled description of claim act."

The **Food, Drug, and Cosmetic Act (FDCA)**, which was created largely in response to the Sulfanilamide Disaster, helped ensure drugs being distributed were safe and fulfilled the reported claim of strength, purity, and quality. The act prohibited the distribution of any drug that was not considered safe by the Food and Drug Administration (FDA). However, the FDCA did not require substances to be effective. Through this act, the FDA was given the power to allow or deny a company to distribute a drug.

Durham-Humphrey Amendment of 1952

RECALL TIP

To help remember what the Durham-Humphrey Amendment did, remember its acronym DHA. "D" represents distinguished, "h" represents harmful, and "a" represents application. Now when you think about DHA, you remember Durham-Humphrey Amendment and "distinguished harmful application."

The **Durham-Humphrey Amendment (DHA)**, which is also known as the prescription drug amendment, separated drugs into two categories: legend drugs (prescription drugs) and over-the-counter drugs (OTC). The act specified that all drugs new to the market can only be distributed to patients through prescriptions, but eventually may be changed to OTC status. In addition, prescription medication bottles must carry a legend (or label) stating that the medication can only be dispensed with a prescription. The DHA also prohibited prescription drugs from being refilled without the consent of the doctor or prescriber.

Kefauver-Harris Amendment of 1962

The **Kefauver-Harris Amendment (KHA)** became part of the FDCA to institute higher safety measures for drugs approved by the FDA. Manufactures became responsible for Good Manufacturing Processes (GMP), which required them to prove both the safety and effectiveness of drugs in clinical trials before the FDA would grant permission for marketing and distribution. If a drug is approved by the FDA for sale in the United States, the drug is considered safe and effective when taken properly. In addition, KHA established definitive procedures for new drug applications (NDA) as well as investigational drugs.

Controlled Substances Act of 1970

The **Controlled Substances Act (CSA)** is part of the Comprehensive Drug Abuse Prevention and Control Act. The CSA was designed to help regulate drug use by creating rules and regulations for record keeping and dispensing, and requiring firms that handle controlled substances to register with the DEA. The CSA also organized controlled substances into a system of schedules based on the potential for abuse.

- Schedule I: Drugs with no medical use and a high potential for abuse, such as heroin and LSD.

- Schedule II: Drugs with a medical use and a high potential for abuse, such as morphine and methamphetamine. If this type of drug is abused, it may lead to severe dependence. No refills are allowed.
- Schedule III: Drugs with a medical use and a potential for abuse, such as codeine and hydrocodone. If this type of drug is abused, it may lead to moderate dependence. Patient may receive up to 5 refills in 6 months.
- Schedule IV: Drugs with medical use and a low potential for abuse, such as diphenoxylate and oxazepam. If this type of drug is abused, it may lead to limited dependence. Patient may receive up to 5 refills in 6 months.
- Schedule V: Drugs with a medical use and a low potential for abuse, such as OTC cough syrups that contain codeine (Phenergan). If this type of drug is abused, it may lead to limited dependence. Patient may receive as many refills as their physician deems appropriate.

> **RECALL TIP**
> To help you remember how drug schedules are organized, think about how you create your own daily schedule. All you need to do is prioritize. Generally, you put the most important task, or in this case the most potential for abuse, first. This item is number one in your priority list. As you go down the priority list, the potential for abuse decreases.

The Poison Prevention Packaging Act of 1970

> **RECALL TIP**
> To help remember what the Controlled Substances Act is all about, remember the act's acronym, CSA. "C" represents created, "S" represents schedules for, and "a" represents abuse. Now, CSA stands for Controlled Substances Act, but it also stands for "created schedules for abuse."

The **Poison Prevention Packaging Act (PPPA)** was created to reduce accidental poisonings. Included in this act are requirements for child-resistant closures on prescription and OTC drugs intended for oral use, as well as a provision requiring manufacturers to include package inserts with certain drugs. The few exemptions to the act include cardiac medications and single dose sizes. The PPPA was originally enforced by the FDA but was later transferred to the Consumer Product Safety Commission when the agency was created in 1973.

The Drug Listing Act of 1972

The **Drug Listing Act** was established to create a list of marketed drugs for the FDA, which would assist with enforcing federal safety laws. All manufacturers or firms that repackage drugs, including foreign firms, are required to register with the FDA. Registered firms are assigned registration numbers that are formatted using the National Drug Code numbering system.

The National Drug Code (NDC) numbering system is a coded system created to identify a drug by simply looking at the code on the label. The code is made up of 10 characters and numbers which are broken up into three segments, either 4:3:3 or 4:4:2.

- Segment 1: identifies the product manufacturer or distributer
- Segment 2: identifies the product code, strength, and dosage form
- Segment 3: identifies package sizes and types

The Orphan Drug Act of 1983

The **Orphan Drug Act** is a special program created by the FDA to speed up the approval process for new medications intended to help people with urgent needs. The FDA created the program to help develop and market treatments for rare diseases (diseases with fewer than 200,000 cases), such as AIDS and Tourette syndrome. To encourage researchers to participate, incentives include grants, protocol assistance by the FDA, and special tax credits. If a drug is approved under the act, the manufacturer gets exclusive marketing rights for seven years.

Prescription Drug Marketing Act of 1987

The Prescription Drug Marketing Act implemented new safety measures for prescription drugs in the United States. The goal of the act is to reduce the risk of repackaged, mislabeled, and adulterated substances entering the marketplace. This was done through:

- prohibiting reimportation of drugs by anyone except manufacturers
- enforcing sales restrictions
- regulating sample distribution

Pharmacy Standards

Specific pharmacy standards are created by your state's Board of Pharmacy. These rules, along with applicable federal laws, create the basis of pharmacy practice. State standards may be stricter than federal laws. In this case, pharmacies are required to practice under the more rigid regulations. To find out what your state requires, go online and search for your state's State Board of Pharmacy.

The Omnibus Budget Reconciliation Act of 1990

The Omnibus Budget Reconciliation Act (OBRA 90) required states to develop programs to improve the quality of pharmaceutical care. OBRA also requires pharmacists to perform Drug Utilization Review (DUR). As a result of these programs, patients receive:

- counseling about prescribed and OTC medications
- warnings about potential allergy interactions
- techniques for self-monitoring drug therapy

Patient Self-Determination Act of 1990

RECALL TIP

Use the phrase "<u>a</u>head <u>deci</u>sions" to remember the idea behind <u>a</u>dvance <u>d</u>irectives. Advance directives are decisions you make about your care ahead of time. You can have your decision in writing with a living will or entrust someone to carry out your wishes with a durable power of attorney.

The Patient Self-Determination Act requires hospitals to inform patients about their rights and their ability to create an advance directive. There are two types of advance directives:

- *Living will.* This document provides very specific instructions about the type of care a patient chooses in particular circumstances. Wishes regarding life-sustaining treatment, artificial nutrition and hydration, and comfort care can all be decided before a person becomes ill.
- *Durable power of attorney.* This allows a patient to choose a representative to make decisions on the patient's behalf should the patient become incapacitated.

Blanket Consent

Blanket consent is a form that allows a physician to do what he or she thinks is necessary for a patient. It is generally signed at the first meeting between a healthcare provider and a patient, and contains language about how the physician has discussed treatment with the patient and the patient has had the opportunity to ask questions.

Pharmacy Best Practices

According to the American Pharmacists Association, the goal of the pharmacy is to responsibly assist society in the use of medication, devices, and services in an effort to achieve an optimum outcome. To do this, pharmacists need to follow specific guidelines and practices when handling and storing controlled substances.

Checking for Prescription Errors

Prescription errors can have deadly consequences. When filling a prescription, it's a good idea to take the following precautions.

- Check the original order against the label, against the bottle of medication before filling, and before filling the vial and labeling.
- Verify the route and dose that the physician ordered with what you prepared.
- Check when and how the patient should take the medication.
- Document the procedure in the patient's medical records: note the date, time, drug, dose, route, site, result/tolerance, and patient education.
- Verify the name on the physician's order.

Ordering and Dispensing Controlled Substances

Since controlled substances have the potential to be abused, pharmacies must abide by requirements regarding the ordering and dispensing of these drugs. For a pharmacist to order, receive, handle, or dispense a controlled substance, the pharmacy must be registered with the DEA and have a DEA registration number. You'll learn more about DEA registrations numbers in Chapter 10: *Dispensing Medications*. Prescription orders also have requirements that must be met before the prescription can be filled. The following prescription requirements pertain to orders for controlled substances in all schedule categories:

- date of issue
- full name and address of the patient
- the drug name, strength, dosage form, and quantity prescribed
- directions for use
- full name, address, and DEA number for the prescriber
- the signature of the prescriber, for written orders
- For Schedule II substances, a written or typed order with the prescriber's signature is required. In an emergency, a physician may also phone in a prescription, but he or she must provide a hard copy of the prescription within 7 days.

Transferring Prescriptions of Non-Controlled Substances

In order to transfer non-controlled substances between pharmacies, pharmacies must follow these specific rules:

1. The prescription transfer can only take place between licensed pharmacies, and the transferring pharmacist must record the following information in the patient medication record system:
   - a copy of the prescription has been issued
   - the name and address of the pharmacy and pharmacist that the prescription was transferred to

2. The pharmacist receiving the prescription must do the following:
   - write "transfer" on the patient's prescription
   - include all required information on the prescription, such as the patient's information and the prescriber's information, along with the name of the transferor pharmacist

3. Once a prescription is transferred, the original pharmacy can no longer refill the prescription.

4. If pharmacies use a common electronic database for prescription recordkeeping, a patient can refill a prescription at any participating pharmacy.

Record Keeping

Pharmacies must follow specific record-keeping requirements for maintaining controlled substances.

- Pharmacies must keep track of the receipt and delivery of all controlled substances, no matter their schedule.
- Controlled substances must be inventoried every 2 years.
- Schedule II drugs must be singled out due to the potential for abuse. For a prescriber to obtain a controlled substance from a pharmacy for office use, the prescriber or pharmacist must order the drug using DEA Form 222. Copies 1 and 2 of the form need to be forwarded to the drug wholesaler, with the carbon paper intact.
- For drugs in other schedules, pharmacies only need to keep the invoice to document receipt.

Storing Controlled Substances

Since controlled substances have the potential for addiction and harm, federal regulations require that controlled substances must be stored in a secure location with strictly limited access. In addition, controlled substances can never be left unattended, and inventory should be limited.

Generally, Schedule II drugs should be stored separately from other Scheduled drugs. However, if the drugs are stored in a community setting, Schedule II can be dispersed throughout the other inventory. Here are other approved and prohibited storage methods:

Approved storage methods include:

- Safes and steels cabinets that are bolted to the floor or wall
- Locking storage drawers that are inaccessible from other drawers

Prohibited storage methods include:

- Portable storage containers
- Corridor storage areas

Legal Implications

When controlled substances are abused, they have the potential to be fatal. Because of this, there are consequences for violating regulations or willfully altering records.

If a pharmacy violates the CSA or DEA regulations, the DEA has the right to seek criminal charges, monetary fines, and/or revoke, suspend, or deny the pharmacy's controlled substance registration or a pharmacist's license.

Similarly, if a pharmacy is caught altering records, it is considered fraud, and the consequences may be the same as violating federal regulations. Check you state's Board of Pharmacy for any additional laws and consequences.

Chapter Summary

- Pharmacology is enforced legally by laws and ethically by peers, professional organizations, and the community.
- Personal information and account numbers are confidential.
- Confidential information can only be released under written consent of the patient, by subpoena, and in cases of mandatory reporting.
- The Food, Drug, and Cosmetic Act ensured drugs were safe and claims made about ingredients were accurate.
- The Durham-Humphrey's Amendment established prescription and over-the-counter drugs.
- The Kefauver-Harris Amendment required manufacturers to prove the safety and effectiveness of drugs.
- The Controlled Substance Act categorized drugs based on potential for abuse and regulated the record keeping and dispensing of controlled substances.
- The Poison Prevention Packaging Act implemented safety closures on drugs to reduce accidental poisonings.
- The Drug Listing Act created a list of marketed drugs for the FDA.
- The National Drug Code numbering system is used to identify drugs by simply looking at the code on the label.
- The Orphan Drug Act was created by the FDA to speed up the approval process for medications for people suffering from rare diseases who have urgent needs.
- The Prescription Drug Marketing Act helped reduce the risk of prepackaged, mislabeled, and adulterated substances from entering the marketplace.
- State pharmacy standards may be stricter than federal laws; pharmacists must follow the more rigid standards.
- OBRA 90 improved the quality of pharmaceutical care through patient education and appropriate practice.
- The Patient Self-Determination Act requires hospitals to inform patients about their healthcare rights and ability to create an advance directive.
- Blanket consent allows a physician to do what he or she thinks is necessary when treating a patient.
- To help prevent prescription errors, check the prescription order, label, and medication storage container for accuracy.
- Pharmacies must be registered with the DEA to order, receive, handle, or dispense a controlled substance.
- Pharmacies must follow specific rules in order to transfer a prescription. Participating pharmacies must be licensed and keep track of all necessary information.
- Controlled substances must be inventoried every two years.
- Controlled substances must be locked in a secure cabinet. In addition, controlled substances can never be left unattended, and inventory for controlled substances should be limited.
- If a pharmacy violates the CSA or DEA regulations, the DEA has the right to seek criminal charges, monetary fines, and/or revoke, suspend, or deny the pharmacy's controlled substance registration or a pharmacist's license.
- If a pharmacy is caught altering records, it is considered fraud, and the consequences may be the same as violating federal regulations.

PRACTICE TEST QUESTIONS

Law and Ethics

1. Which amendment or act is also known as the prescription drug amendment?
   a. Kefauver-Harris Amendment
   b. Omnibus Budget Reconciliation Act
   c. Durham-Humphrey Amendment
   d. Poison Prevention Packaging Act

2. Which of the following is considered "confidential" information?
   a. Directory information
   b. License number
   c. Country of origin
   d. Marital status

3. Which organization enforces the Poison Prevention Packaging Act?
   a. The Council of Health-System Pharmacists
   b. Food and Drug Administration
   c. Drug Enforcement Administration
   d. Consumer Product Safety Commission

4. What is a safe and effective drug?
   a. A medication classified as a Schedule V controlled substance
   b. A drug approved by the FDA for sale in the United States
   c. A medication that prevents pregnancy
   d. A drug that has no side effects

5. The Kefauver-Harris Amendment of 1962 requires drug manufacturers prove to the FDA:
   a. the effectiveness of their products before marketing them.
   b. that household substances packaged for consumers use child-resistant packaging.
   c. that drugs which cannot be used safely without medical supervision, be labeled for sale and be dispensed by a prescription of an authorized prescriber.
   d. All of the above

6. When completing DEA form 222 to obtain Schedule II medications, which requirement must be met?
   a. Copies one and two must be forwarded to the wholesaler, with the carbon paper intact.
   b. The form must be handwritten in pencil.
   c. More than one item must be ordered per line.
   d. Suppliers must accept and fill an order even if it has errors and erasures.

7. Which federal law ensured that drugs being distributed were safe and fulfilled reported claims?
   a. Controlled Substances Act
   b. Omnibus Budget Reconciliation Act
   c. Food, Drug, and Cosmetic Act
   d. Durham-Humphrey Act

8. Which law requires pharmacists to counsel patients on new medications?
   a. Durham-Humphrey's Amendment
   b. Comprehensive Drug Abuse Prevention and Control Act
   c. Prescription Drug Marketing Act
   d. Omnibus Budget Reconciliation Act

9. What is the purpose of the Orphan Drug Act?
   a. Stops the use of drugs without a prescription in animals
   b. Allows drug companies to bypass lengthy testing to treat persons who have a rare disease
   c. Ensures safety and effectiveness of manufacturing practices
   d. Applies stricter rules concerning controlled substances sales and distribution

10. The best time to check for errors on a prescription while filling is:
    a. when the order is first received, during filling, and after filling.
    b. while filling the order, after filling, and when handing the medication to the patient.
    c. when checking the original order against the label, against the stock bottle before filling, and before filling the vial and labeling.
    d. before applying the label, before applying the auxiliary labels, and before giving the final product to the pharmacist to check.

11. Which of the following statements identifies "blanket consent"?
    a. A separate consent form must be signed for each individual procedure.
    b. The consent outlines many items of routine care and/or information and is signed on the first encounter with a healthcare provider.
    c. The physician regarding risks, side effects and benefits must give detailed information.
    d. It is used in case of emergency.

12. The middle segment of a national drug code represents which of the following product elements?

   a. Product code, strength, and dosage form
   b. Package size, manufacturer, and strength
   c. Dosage form and manufacturer
   d. Package size and product strength

13. In a court of law, the intentional altering of records will result in a charge of:

   a. felony.
   b. misdemeanor.
   c. forgery.
   d. fraud.

14. The Patient Self-Determination Act, a federal law relating to end-of-life decisions for patients with terminal illnesses, requires two different documents under federal law. The two documents are called:

   a. Emergency Consent and Durable Power of Attorney.
   b. Advance Directive and Specific Consent.
   c. Durable Power of Attorney and Living Will
   d. General Consent and Guardian Directive.

15. Which of the following statements about transfer requirements is TRUE regarding refillable non-controlled substances?

   a. Prescriptions can be refilled three times between non-related, non-networked pharmacies.
   b. Prescriptions can be refilled as many times as the prescription is refillable if the pharmacies share an electronic real-time database.
   c. Prescriptions can be refilled as often as the patient and prescriber agree.
   d. Prescription refills are up to the discretion of the pharmacist.

16. Controlled substances for office use can be obtained by a prescriber:

   a. through DEA order form 222.
   b. with a prescription marked "For Office Use Only."
   c. per a phone order.
   d. by visiting a pharmacy and showing proper identification.

17. A controlled substance inventory must be conducted by a pharmacy:

   a. every year.
   b. every two years.
   c. every three years.
   d. every four years.

18. What action can be taken by the DEA if it feels a pharmacy has violated CSA or DEA regulations?

   a. It may seek criminal penalties.
   b. It may seek civil monetary fines.
   c. It may revoke, suspend, or deny the pharmacy's controlled substances registration.
   d. All of the above

19. Which statement below is TRUE regarding the Controlled Substances Act?

   a. The Act establishes a system of schedules classifying drugs by their potential for abuse.
   b. The Act requires the registration of individuals and organizations that handle controlled substances.
   c. The Act requires strict recordkeeping of controlled substances inventories.
   d. All of the above

21. A physician prescribes Percocet for a patient going home after abdominal surgery. The patient eventually runs out of the drug and calls the pharmacy for a refill. The technician explains to the patient that:

   a. This medication can only be filled twice.
   b. This medication has an unlimited amount of refills.
   c. This medication will need another prescription from the physician, because it does not allow refills.
   d. This medication must be refilled within 30 days of the first prescription.

22. Schedule IV controlled substances can be refilled:

   a. As many times as the provider allows.
   b. 5 times in 6 months.
   c. Twice.
   d. Zero times; refills are not allowed.

3

Medical Abbreviations and Terminology

Test Topics

After completing this chapter, you should be able to demonstrate knowledge of the following:

1. Pharmaceutical and medical abbreviations and terminology
2. Generic and brand names of pharmaceuticals
3. Therapeutic equivalence

Test Terms

- **brand name** the name a manufacturer assigns to a drug
- **capsule** a pill-like shell that contains a liquid or powder form of medication; dissolves when it reaches the stomach, releasing the medication
- **elixir** thin and watery medication that may contain alcohol
- **generic name** the official name assigned to a drug
- **hypothyroidism** condition that occurs when the body does not produce adequate amounts of thyroid hormone
- **hyperthyroidism** condition that occurs when the body produces excessive amounts of thyroid hormone
- **mechanism of action** the way a drug works
- **pharmacology** the study of drugs and how they work in therapeutic use
- **pharmaceutical equivalent** medications that have identical active ingredients, dosages, and routes of administration
- **potentiation** the process of one drug becoming more effective through the simultaneous administration of another drug
- **solution** a liquid form of medication that contains medications in a water base
- **suspension** form of a medication that is mixed into a liquid but not fully dissolved
- **syrup** a thicker, sugar-based liquid form of medication
- **tablets** form of medication that is a solid, such as a pill
- **therapeutic effect** the intended effect in the treatment of a symptom or illness
- **tincture** a total alcohol solution

Familiarity with a variety of medical terms and abbreviations will be key to your success as a pharmacy technician. In addition, recognizing the corresponding generic names for commonly prescribed brand name medications is another important responsibility. You will also need to be knowledgeable about the language used to express drug classifications.

Basic Terms

Pharmacology is the study of drugs and how they work in therapeutic use. The amount of the drug that is administered in a given case is the dose. The way a drug works is known as the **mechanism of action**, and its intended effect in the treatment of a symptom or illness is called the **therapeutic effect**.

Often times, drugs have unwanted or unexpected side effects. For example, certain blood pressure medications may cause dizziness. With **potentiation**, the effect of one drug is increased through the simultaneous administration of another drug.

Forms of Oral Medication

Medications may be administered in a variety of different forms. In general, medication forms fall into one of three categories: solid, liquid, and semisolid. Some solid dosage forms include:

- **tablets**: the solid, pill form of a medication.
- **capsules**: pill-like shells that contain a liquid or powder form of medication. The shell dissolves when it reaches the stomach, releasing the medication.
- caplets
- lozenges/troches
- transdermal patches

Liquid dosage forms include:

- **suspensions**: medications mixed into a liquid but not dissolved. For this reason, suspensions usually carry the direction "Shake Well." Flavored suspensions are often used to administer medications to children, who may have difficulty swallowing tablets.
- **solutions**: another liquid form of medication that contains medications in a water base.
- **elixirs**: thin and watery medications that may contain alcohol.
- **syrups**: a thicker, sugar-based liquid form of medication.
- **tinctures**: total alcohol solutions.
- emulsions
- sprays
- inhalents and aerosol enemas

Semisolid dosage forms include:

- creams
- lotions
- ointments
- gels
- pastes
- suppositories
- powders
- injectables

Generic and Brand Name Drugs

Pharmaceuticals have two names: the generic name and the brand name. The **generic name** is the official name assigned to a drug. It refers to the drug's active ingredient. The **brand name** (or trade name) is the name the manufacturer gives to the drug. For example, setraline is the generic name for the widely distributed brand-name antidepressant Zoloft. Some drugs have more than one brand name because they are manufactured and sold by multiple pharmaceutical companies. Drugs that have identical active ingredients, dosages, and routes of administration are said to have **pharmaceutical equivalence.**

Medical Abbreviations for Time and Frequency

RECALL TIP

Knowledge of the Latin words and phrases from which many medical abbreviations are derived may make it easier for you to identify the meaning behind the letters. For example:

• *ante* = before (A)
• *post* = after (P)
• *quaque* = every (Q)

To accurately interpret a prescription, you will need to understand and decode a variety of medical abbreviations. Many of these medical abbreviations relate to the time and frequency with which a given medication is to be dispensed. They are based on Latin phrases, thus their meanings are not always obvious without prior knowledge. The following table summarizes common medical abbreviations.

Common Abbreviations

Abbreviation	Meaning	Abbreviation	Meaning
a	before	pm	after noon
ac	before meals	po	oral or by mouth
am	before noon	pr	per rectum
ad	right ear	prn	as needed
as	left ear	q	every
au	both ears	qd	every day
bid	twice a day	qh	every hour
d	day	qod	every other day
gtt	drops	q2h	every 2 hours
h	hour	qid	four times a day
hs	at hour of sleep (bedtime)	ss	one-half
noc	night	stat	immediately
od	right eye	supp	suppository
os	left eye	tid	three times a day
ou	both eyes	tiw	three times a week
p	after	wk	week
pc	after meals	yr	year

Commonly Prescribed Drugs and Classifications

Pharmaceuticals are often classified, or categorized, based on both how they affect the body and what illnesses or symptoms they typically treat. Familiarity with the brand and generic names of commonly prescribed medications, in addition to their classifications, is vital to your work as a pharmacy technician.

Drugs that Treat Endocrine System Disorders

The endocrine system is comprised of glands that produce hormones. These hormones regulate the body's growth and metabolism. As a result, drugs that treat disorders of the endocrine system often affect how the body produces hormones.

Antidiabetics

RECALL TIP

Use the acronym DIG—Diabetes, Insulin, Glucagon—to remember the association between diabetes and the hormones insulin and glucagon.

Glucagon and insulin are hormones that regulate carbohydrate/sugar metabolism. They are secreted by the pancreas. In people with diabetes, the pancreas does not produce or properly use insulin.

Oral antidiabetics are a class of drugs that work to lower elevated blood sugar in people with diabetes by stimulating the release of insulin and/or preventing the release of glucose. Some medications, such as metaformin, can also be used to increase the body's sensitivity to insulin. The following table provides examples of commonly prescribed oral antidiabetics.

Classification: Oral Antidiabetics	
Generic Name	**Brand Name**
pioglitazone	Actos
glimepiride	Amaryl
rosiglitazone	Avandia
glipizide	Glucotrol
tolbutamide	Orinase
metformin	Glucophage

Hormone Replacements

RECALL TIP

Both "thyroid" and "iodine" contain long "I" sounds when pronounced. Use this similarity to remember that iodine helps the body produce thyroid hormones.

Iodine is a naturally occurring element that is used by the body to produce thyroid hormones. It is found in seafood, as well as in iodized salt. In some instances, the body may not produce adequate amounts of thyroid hormone, leading to a condition called **hypothyroidism**.

In these cases a thyroid replacement may be prescribed. These drugs correct the deficiency of the thyroid hormones. The following table highlights common thyroid replacements.

Thyroid Replacements	
Generic Name	**Brand Name**
levothyroxine	Levoxyl, Levothroid, Synthroid
liothyronine	Cytomel

Drugs That Treat Respiratory Disorders

Respiratory drugs are used to treat conditions such as asthma, allergy symptoms, and coughing and congestion. There are several different classes of respiratory drugs.

Bronchodilators

Bronchodilators are drugs that dilate the muscular walls of the bronchi. They are often prescribed to treat asthma.

- Beta 2 agonists are a type of bronchodilator that are typically inhaled and act rapidly. Also referred to as beta adrenergic drugs, these medications work by causing epinephrine to stimulate the Beta-2 receptors in the respiratory tract. This, in turn, relaxes smooth muscles and leads to bronchodilation.
- Xanthines work as bronchodilators that work by relaxing the smooth muscles involved in respiration.
- Acetylcholine (ACH) is a neurotransmitter that plays a key role in muscular movement. Anticholinergic are drugs that block the action of acetylcholine, thus working as bronchodilators.

Corticosteroids

Corticosteroids are another classification of drugs sometimes prescribed to ease respiratory symptoms. They work by reducing inflammation. Corticosteroids may also be prescribed to control inflammation associated with immunological disorders. The following table lists some major corticosteroids.

Corticosteroids	
Generic Name	**Brand Name**
hydrocortisone	Cortef
prednisone	Deltasone
betamethasone	Diprosone
prednisolone	Pediapred
methylprednisolone	SoluMedrol

Antihistamines

Histamine is a compound in the body that is released by injured cells during allergic reactions and inflammation. It causes constrictions of the bronchial smooth muscle and dilation of blood vessels. Antihistamines are drugs that neutralize or inhibit the effects of histamine. They are often prescribed to treat allergy symptoms.

Other Respiratory Drugs

Other respiratory drugs are used to treat symptoms such as coughing and congestion. Antitussives reduce coughing by acting on the nerve receptors within the respiratory tract And the medulla in the brain's cough reflex center. A decongestant is a drug that reduces congestion and swelling of membranes, such as those of the nose and eustachian tube after infection. They decrease mucous production. Decongestants such as pseudoephedrine (Sudafed), phenylephrine (Neo-Synephrine 4-Hr, 4-Way Fast Acting, Afrin Children's), and oxymetolazine (Afrin, Dristan) are also called alpha adrenergic drugs. Alpha adrenergic drugs affect the alpha-adrenergic receptors in the nose. They cause constriction of the blood vessels in this area, which relieves congestion through an anti-inflammatory effect.

See the following table for examples of commonly prescribed respiratory drugs.

Respiratory Drugs			
Generic Name	Brand Name	Classification	Use
oxymetazoline	Afrin Topical Decongestant, Dristan 12-Hr Nasal Spray	decongestant	cold
ipratropium	Atrovent	bronchodilator (anticholinergic)	asthma, COPD
triamcinolone acetonide	Azmacort	inhaled corticosteroid	asthma
beclomethasone	Beclovent, Vanceril	inhaled corticosteroid	asthma
diphenhyrdramine	Benadryl	antihistamine	cold, allergy
loratadine	Claritin	antihistamine	allergy
phenylephrine	Neo-Synephrine 4-Hr, 4-Way Fast Acting, Afrin Children's	decongestant	cold
pseudoephedrine	Sudafed	decongestant	cold
benzonatate	Tessalon	antitussive	cough
theophylline	Theodur, Bronkody	bronchodilator (xanthine)	asthma
levalbuterol	Xopenex	bronchodilator (beta 2 agonist)	asthma
cetirizine	Zyrtec	antihistamine	allergy

Drugs That Affect the Cardiovascular System

The table on page TK summarizes several types of cardiovascular drugs:

- Beta blockers treat hypertension and angina pectoris by blocking responses to sympathetic adrenergic nerve activity. In addition, some beta blockers, including propanolol (Inderal) are used to treat migraines and anxiety.
- Diuretics (e.g. Microzine) also treat hypertension. They work by increasing the secretion of urine, which means excess sodium and water are eliminated.
- ACE inhibitors (e.g. Enalapril) prevent the conversion of AI enzymes into AII enzymes, which are vasoconstrictors.
- AII Receptor Antagonists (e.g. Diovan) block the effects of the AII enzyme at receptor sites.
- Antihyperlipidemics (e.g. Liptor) inhibit the synthesis of HMG-CoA Reductase, which is needed to produce cholesterol

Cardiovascular Drugs

Generic Name	Brand Name	Classification	Use
hydrochlorothiazide (HCTZ)	Aquazide H, Hyrdrodiuril, Microzine	diuretic	hypertension
propanolol	Inderal	beta blocker	hypertension, migraines, anxiety
enalapril	Vasotec	ACE inhibitor	hypertension
valsartan	Diovan	AII receptor antagonist	hypertension
atorvastatin	Lipitor	Antihyperlipidemic	high cholesterol

Drugs That Treat Musculoskeletal Disorders

Muscle relaxants are drugs prescribed to reduce pain associated with injuries. In addition, they may be used to treat symptoms associated with diseases such as multiple sclerosis and cerebral palsy. For example, baclofen (Lioresal) is used to treat reversible spasticity and spinal cord lesions. Diazepam (Valium) is considered by many to be the "best" muscle relaxant because of its short acting calming effects as well as its antispasmodic properties. However, this drug should be used with caution, as it has a high potential for addiction and abuse. See the following table for a list of common muscle relaxants.

Muscle Relaxants

Generic Name	Brand Name
dantrolene sodium	Dantrium
diazepam	Valium
cyclobenzaprine hydrochloride	Flexeril
baclofen	Lioresal
orphenadrine	Norflex
chlorzoxazone	Paraflex
methocarbamol	Robaxin
carisoprodol	Soma
diazepam	Valium
tizanidine hydrochloride	Zanaflex

Drugs That Treat Nervous System Disorders

The nervous system, comprised of billions of nerve cells, is tremendously complex. Drugs that treat disorders of the nervous system often affect neurotransmitters, chemicals that pass impulses between nerves.

- Anticonvulsants are drugs that prevent or lessen convulsions. Convulsions are abnormal, involuntary muscle contractions. Anticonvulsants are often prescribed to treat seizure disorders. The table on page TK lists commonly prescribed anticonvulsants.

- Several different classifications of drugs are used to treat pain. Some, such as NSAIDs, are anti-inflammatory agents that reduce swelling and can relieve mild-to-moderate pain. Other kinds of drugs, such as narcotics, can be used to treat more severe forms of pain by dulling pain receptors in the brain.

- Stimulants speed up the activity of the nervous system. Methylphenidate (Ritalin) is a mild stimulant used to treat ADHD. It works in part by blocking the reuptake of dopamine (DA).

- Dopaminergics are drugs that act like the naturally occurring neurotransmitter dopamine. (DA), which plays a key role in movement and coordination. They may be used to treat diseases such as Parkinson's, which is characterized by a deficiency of dopamine in the brain and thus, difficulties with movement.

- Anticholinesterase drugs, including erdophonium (Tenlison), treat diseases such as myasthenia gravis, which are characterized by muscle weakness. They are called anticholinesterase drugs because they block the action of acetylcholinesterase, an enzyme that breaks down ACH.

- Antidepressants affect the concentration of neurotransmitters including serotonin and norepinephrine in the brain. One type of antidepressant, selective serotonin reuptake inhibitors (SSRIs), works by blocking the reuptake of the neurotransmitter serotonin in the brain. Serotonin plays a significant role in both sleep and feelings of emotional arousal.

See the table on page TK for a list of additional drugs that affect the nervous system.

RECALL TIP
Use alliteration to help you remember that serotonin plays a role in regulating sleep.

Anticonvulsants	
Generic Name	**Brand Name**
divalproex	Depakote
gabapentin	Neurontin
carbamazepine	Tegretol
topiramate	Topamax
ethosuximide	Zarontin

Drugs That Affect the Nervous System			
Generic Name	**Brand Name**	**Classification**	**Use**
naproxen	Aleve	NSAID	mild-to-moderate pain, migraines
oxycodone	Oxycontin	narcotic	moderate-to-severe pain
bromocriptine	Parlodel	dopaminergic	Parkinson's

(continued)

Drugs That Affect the Nervous System *(continued)*			
Generic Name	**Brand Name**	**Classification**	**Use**
methylphenidate	Ritalin	CNS stimulant	ADHD
edrophonium	Tensilon	anticholinesterase	myasthenia gravis
setraline	Zoloft	antidepressant (SSRI)	depression
Triazolam	Halcion	benzodiazepine	insomnia

Chapter Summary

- The way in which a drug treats a symptom or illness is its therapeutic effect. Pharmaceuticals have generic names, which refer to their active ingredient, and brand names, which are given to them by the pharmaceutical companies that manufacture and market them.
- Prescriptions often include medical abbreviations to express the time and frequency of dosing.
- Antidiabetics and hormone replacements are types of drugs used to treat endocrine disorders.
- Drugs that relieve the symptoms of respiratory disorders include bronchodilators, corticosteroids, antihistamines, antitussives, and decongestants.
- Beta blockers and diuretics treat hypertension; muscle relaxants ease muscoskeletal pain.
- Anticonvulsants, stimulants, dopaminergics, and antidepressants are examples of drugs that affect the nervous system.

PRACTICE TEST QUESTIONS

Medical Abbreviations and Terminology

1. Liquids that carry the direction "Shake Well" are usually:
   a. elixirs.
   b. syrups.
   c. solutions.
   d. suspensions.

2. A semisolid dosage form whose base contains more water and penetrates well into the skin are:
   a. creams.
   b. ointments.
   c. lotions.
   d. emulsions.

3. A type of dosage form that has a sugar-based solution that the medication dissolves into is called a(n):

   a. elixir.
   b. syrup.
   c. aerosol.
   d. suspension.

4. A types of dosage form composed of a gelatin container and comes in different sizes is called a:
   a. caplet.
   b. lozenge.
   c. troche.
   d. capsule.

5. A type of liquid dosage form that contains dissolved medication in an alcohol base or water is called a(n):
   a. elixir.
   b. syrup.
   c. suspension.
   d. solution.

6. The brand name for glimepiride is:
   a. Actos.
   b. Amaryl.
   c. Avandia.
   d. Orinase.

7. Potentiation:
   a. describes a side effect.
   b. is the joint action of a drug.
   c. increases the effect of another drug.
   d. causes a therapeutic effect.

8. The medical abbreviation for 4 times a day is:
   a. QID.
   b. BID.
   c. TID.
   d. QD.

9. The generic name for Azmacort is:
   a. cetirizine.
   b. triamcinolone acetonide.
   c. levalbuterol.
   d. beclomethasone.

10. Decongestants are prescribed to:
    a. treat allergic rhinitis.
    b. eliminate airway obstruction.
    c. treat asthma.
    d. decrease mucous production.

11. Theophylline is classified as a(n):
    a. antihistamine.
    b. anticholinergic.
    c. beta 2 agonist.
    d. bronchodilator.

12. The element from the diet that is used by the body to produce thyroid hormone is:
    a. aluminum.
    b. sodium.
    c. iodine.
    d. calcium.

13. The generic name for SoluMedrol is:
    a. methylprednisolone.
    b. prednisone.
    c. prednisolone.
    d. betamethasone.

14. Deltasone, Cortef, and Pediapred are classified as:
    a. Therapeutic corticosteroids.
    b. Hormones to treat osteoporosis.
    c. Glucocorticoids.
    d. Thyroid replacement.

15. All the following are brand names of synthetic levothyroxine except:
    a. Levoxyl.
    b. Cytomel.
    c. Levothroid.
    d. Synthroid.

16. The drug used to treat reversible spasticity or spinal cord lesions is:
    a. tizanadine.
    b. diazepam.
    c. baclofen.
    d. orphenadrine.

17. The neurotransmitter involved with sleep and emotional arousal is:
    a. acetylcholine.
    b. dopamine.
    c. norephinephrine.
    d. serotonin.

18. The brand name for methocarbamol is:
    a. Dantrium.
    b. Robaxin.
    c. Flexeril.
    d. Zanaflex.

19. What drug is considered to be the "best" muscle relaxer?
    a. Soma
    b. Valium
    c. Lioresal
    d. Flexeril

20. The generic name for Norflex is:
    a. chlorzoxazone.
    b. carisoprodol.
    c. orphenadrine.
    d. baclofen.

21. Pseudoephedrine, phenylephrine, and oxymetolazine are classified as:
    a. alpha adrenergic drugs.
    b. beta adrenergic drugs.
    c. alpha cholinergic drugs.
    d. muscle relaxants.

22. All of the following are drugs used to treat diabetes except:
    a. Metformin.
    b. Glipizide.
    c. Glucagon.
    d. HCTZ.

23. The medical abbreviation for after meals is:
    a. AC.
    b. HS.
    c. PO.
    d. PC.

24. The generic name for Allegra is:
    a. oxymetazoline.
    b. fenxofenadine.
    c. clemastine.
    d. trimeprazine.

25. The generic name for Neurontin is:
    a. topiramate.
    b. gabapentin.
    c. carbamazepine.
    d. ethosuximide.

26. The generic name for Inderal is:
    a. benzonatate.
    b. diphenhydramine.
    c. propranolol.
    d. metoclopramide.

27. Tegretol and Zarontin are classified as:
    a. seizure medications.
    b. blocking agents for the reuptake of DA.
    c. anticholinergic agents.
    d. immunosuppressants.

28. The medical abbreviation "ac" means:
    a. after meals.
    b. bedtime.
    c. as needed.
    d. before meals.

29. The generic name for Tensilon is:
    a. methylphenidate.
    b. edrophonium.
    c. pyridostigmine.
    d. bromocriptine.

4

Anatomy, Physiology, and Disease

Test Topics

After completing this chapter, you should be able to demonstrate knowledge of the following:

1. Anatomy and physiology
2. Epidemiology
3. Risk factors for disease
4. Signs and symptoms of disease states
5. Standard and abnormal laboratory values

Test Terms

- **afferent neurons** neurons that relay information to the CNS
- **Alzheimer disease** progressive neurological disorder that results from the degeneration of the cerebral cortex and hippocampus and low levels of the neurotransmitter acetycholine
- **anatomy** the study of body structure
- **asthma** an inflammatory disorder that affects the bronchial tubes of the lungs, characterized by bronchospasms, airway constriction, mucous membrane swelling, and increased mucus production
- **autonomic nervous system (ANS)** responsible for involuntary control of smooth muscle, cardiac muscle, and glands
- **bradycardia** a heart rate of less than 60 beats per minute
- **central nervous system (CNS)** the brain and spinal chord
- **congestive heart failure (CHF)** condition that results from the heart's inability to pump enough blood to vital parts of the body, often leading to an increase in blood pressure and an excess retention of fluid in the lungs, liver, and other parts of the body
- **coronary artery disease (CAD)** condition affecting the blood vessels that feed the heart muscle, allowing a build-up of plaque inside the vessels that over time causes them to narrow, thicken, and become unable to carry blood to other parts of the body
- **Diabetes** a disorder of the pancreas involving production of insulin
- **disease** anything that upsets the structure or function of a part, organ, or system of the body
- **efferent neurons** neurons that carry information from the CNS to muscles and glands
- **emphysema** a chronic obstructive pulmonary disorder that occurs when the alveoli are permanently enlarged due to exposure to outside irritants like cigarette smoke or air pollution

- **epidemiology** the study of epidemics caused by infectious agents, toxic agents, air pollution, and other health-related phenomena
- **master gland** the pituitary gland, which releases the hormones that affect how other glands work
- **osteoporosis** a bone disorder in which bones become fragile due to a lack of normal calcium salt deposits and a decrease in bone protein
- **parasympathetic nervous system** part of the ANS, includes fibers that originate in the brain stem and sacral regions of the spinal cord
- **Parkinson disease** progressive neurologic disorder usually caused by the death of cells in the part of the brain that produces dopamine
- **peripheral nervous system (PNS)** all nerves other than the brain and spinal chord
- **physiology** the study of how the body functions
- **somatic nervous system** responsible for voluntarily control of the skeletal system
- **stroke** brain disorder, also called a cerebrovascular accident, usually caused by a blockage of blood flow to certain areas of brain tissue
- **sympathetic nervous system** part of the ANS, includes fibers that originate in the thoracic and lumbar regions of the spinal cord
- **tachycardia** a heart rate of more than 100 beats per minute

Understanding how health and illness affects people is at the heart of what a pharmacy technician does. In order to perform your job well, you must be aware of the physical and structural makeup of the human body. This will allow you to understand how diseases can disrupt or impair the body's natural functions. Your familiarity with the intricacies of how the body interacts with and defends itself against disease will help you understand the medications you will be dispensing.

The Human Body

Anatomy is the scientific term for the study of body structure. **Physiology** is the term for the study of how the body functions. These two terms, though, are closely related because form and function are intertwined. The human body's makeup is intricately designed for optimum functionality. Anything that upsets the normal structure or working of the body is considered a disease.

The human body has a number of individual systems. Let's review some of the major body systems in more detail.

Integumentary, Skeletal, and Muscular Systems

The most visible and recognizable parts of the body are the skin, bones, and muscles. The body systems that house these parts are the same ones that provide the body's overall structure and act as the body's first line of defense.

- The integumentary system consists of the skin and its associated structures including hair, nails, sweat glands, and oil glands.

- The skeletal system consists of 206 bones and the joints between them—also known as the skeleton. It is the basic framework of the body.
- The muscular system includes skeletal muscles, which protect the organs and maintain a body's posture. This system also includes smooth muscle—which makes up the walls of the organs, and cardiac muscles—which make up the walls of the heart.

Endrocrine System

The endocrine system consists of organs throughout the body, known as glands, which produce hormones that regulate growth, food utilization, and reproduction. The "**master gland**" of the endocrine system is the pituitary gland because it releases the hormones that affect how other glands work. These glands include the thyroid, located in the neck, the pancreas, located in the abdomen, and the adrenals, located on the kidneys.

Cardiovascular System

The cardiovascular system is comprised of the heart and blood vessels that feed valuable substances like oxygen and nutrients to all of the body's tissues. Like any other system in the body, the heart is reliant on several systems interacting with one another. For example, the heart rate is greatly influenced by the nervous system because the autonomic nervous system is responsible for modifying the heart rate. A relatively slow rate of less than 60 beats/minute, also called **bradycardia**, normally occurs during periods of sleep or rest. **Tachycardia**, a heart rate of more than 100 beats/minute, is a normal rate for times of exercise or stress. In either case, the cardiovascular system is working in hand with the nervous system to regulate the heart.

Respiratory System

The respiratory system, which consists of the lungs and all passages that lead to and from them, is responsible for our breathing. It takes in the air we breathe and separates the oxygen from it to pass along through the blood to the heart via the left atrium. Carbon dioxide is, in turn, removed from the tissues and expelled through the lungs.

The Nervous System

The nervous system essentially coordinates all of the systems in the body. Structurally, it is divided into two main components:

- **central nervous system (CNS)**—which consists of the brain and spinal cord
- **peripheral nervous system (PNS)**—which is made up all of the nerves that aren't part of the central nervous system

These two systems interact through highly specialized cells called neurons. The neurons that relay information *to* the CNS are called **afferent neurons**. Neurons that carry information *from* the CNS to muscles and glands are called **efferent neurons**.

In addition to being divided by structural categories, the nervous system is also grouped by functional divisions. These divisions include the **somatic nervous system**, which is responsible for voluntarily control of the skeletal system, and the **autonomic nervous system (ANS)**, which is responsible for involuntary control of smooth muscle, cardiac muscle, and glands. Furthermore, the ANS is subdivided into two systems.

- The **sympathetic nervous system** includes fibers that originate in the thoracic and lumbar regions of the spinal cord. This system contains adrenergic neurons that release epinephrine and norepinephrine.
- The **parasympathetic nervous system** includes fibers that originate in the brain stem and sacral regions of the spinal cord. This system contains cholinergic neurons that release acetylcholine.

Both the sympathetic and parasympathetic systems are controlled in the brain by the hypothalamus. Located in the interbrain, between the cerebral hemispheres and brain stem, the hypothalamus is responsible for most of the body's most vital functions, including the heartbeat, blood vessel contraction, and hormone secretion, just to name a few.

See the following table for a quick review of the functional divisions of the nervous system.

Functional Divisions of the Nervous System		
Division	**Control**	**Effectors**
Somatic nervous system	Voluntary	Skeletal muscle
Autonomic nervous system	Involuntary	Smooth muscle, cardiac muscle, and glands

Epidemiology

Studying anatomy, physiology, and disease on an individual level is important in understanding how the body works. However, to understand how health and disease affects the population as a whole, you must be familiar with **epidemiology**. This methodology of health research is vital to practitioners of preventative medicine who must identify the risk factors of disease.

An epidemiologist specializes in several areas, including:

- epidemics caused by infectious agents
- studying toxic agents, air pollution, and other health-related phenomena
- working with sexually transmitted disease control

Predisposing Causes of Disease

As you know, a **disease** is anything that upsets the structure or function of a part, organ, or system of the body. There are predisposing causes, or risk factors, that increase the likelihood of illness in an individual. Some risk factors include:

- *Age.* Some diseases affect certain age groups more than others.
- *Gender.* Some diseases affect one gender more than the other.
- *Heredity.* People who have a family history of certain diseases have a high probability of inheriting the predisposition to those diseases.
- *Living conditions and habits.* Behavior and environment are key determinants to the state of one's health.

- *Emotional disturbance.* The body's physical structure can sometimes be upset by emotional disturbances, such as stress or anxiety.
- *Physical and chemical damage.* Any physical injury—such as cuts, burns, and fractures—can also lead to infection or degeneration. Exposure to harmful chemicals can also lead to an increase in diseases.
- *Preexisting illness.* People who already suffer from one disease, especially if that disease is chronic, have a greater probability of contracting more diseases.

Disorders by Body System

Diseases and disorders, no matter how they are contracted, can disrupt how organs and systems function and deteriorate their structural integrity. Each of the body's various systems are affected by specific diseases.

The Integumentary System

The following are some types of skin disorders.

- Acne disrupts the sebaceous, or oil, glands that are connected to hair follicles and is found most often in young people. Acne can also be considered an endocrine disease since it also affects hormone-producing glands.
- Cancer of the skin is the most widespread form of cancer that affects people in the United States. Skin cancer development is most associated with exposure to sunlight.
- Viral infections such as herpes simplex virus, which causes cold sores and fever blisters, and shingles, which is caused by the same virus that causes chickenpox in children, affect the skin as well.
- Fungal infections are caused by microorganisms called dermatophytes. Also known as ringworm, these infections are difficult to treat. For example, onychomycosis, which causes thickening, discoloration, and crumbling of the nail bed, requires months of antifungal treatment. Another type of fungal infection is candidiadis, also known as thrush.
- Bacterial skin infections are common and include folliculitis (infection of hair follicles) and erythrasma (which occurs in places where skin touches skin, as between the toes). Most bacterial infections are caused by either *Staphylococcus aureus* or *Stretococcus* and are treated with antibiotics.

The Skeletal System

Bones and joints are particularly susceptible to injury. Athletes, for example, often suffer dislocations or sprains due to the extra stress placed on their extremities. Other skeletal disorders include arthritis (inflammation of the joints) and **osteoporosis**. Osteoporosis is a bone disorder in which bones become fragile due to a lack of normal calcium salt deposits and a decrease in bone protein. People with osteoporosis may experience stress fractures even during the course of normal activity.

The Nervous System

The brain and its associated structures are susceptible to several disorders by infection, injury, and other factors. Below are several disorders of the brain and nervous system.

- **Stroke**, also called a cerebrovascular accident, is the most common form of brain disorder. Strokes are usually caused by a blockage of blood flow to certain areas of brain tissue.

- **Alzheimer disease** results from the degeneration of the cerebral cortex and hippocampus and low levels of the neurotransmitter acetycholine. To date, there are several available drug therapies, though none of them are able to keep the disease from progressing.

- **Parkinson disease** is another progressive neurologic disorder that is usually caused by the death of cells in the part of the brain that produces dopamine. Parkinsonism, like Alzheimer disease, is progressive despite the availability of treatment options.

The Endocrine System

Diabetes is the most common disease that affects the endocrine system. Diabetes typically falls under two main categories.

- **Type I Diabetes**, also called insulin-dependent diabetes mellitus (IDDM) is the less common type, but it is more likely to be fatal. Usually affecting younger patients, type I diabetes results from the body's autoimmune destruction of the pancreas' insulin-producing cells. The blood disorder hyperglycemia is often associated in patients with this diabetes type.

- **Type II Diabetes**, also called non-insulin-dependent diabetes mellitus (NIDDM), is much more common and typically affects overweight adults and children. Sufferers of type II diabetes are still able to produce insulin; however, their body cells are more likely to resist these hormones.

Two other kinds of diabetes are drug-induced diabetes and gestational diabetes. Drug-induced diabetes is not very common, but can occur in patients receiving long-term treatment with lithium salts and in critically ill patients being treated with multiple drugs. Gestational Diabetes occurs in approximately 4% of pregnant women and its cause is unknown. Late in pregnancy, the woman's body is not able to make and use all the insulin it needs, leading to hyperglycemia and causing the pancreas to overproduce insulin.

The Cardiovascular System

There are several disorders associated with the body's cardiovascular system. Among these are the following:

- **Congestive heart failure (CHF)** is a common condition that results from the heart's inability to pump enough blood to vital parts of the body, often leading to an increase in blood pressure and an excess retention of fluid in the lungs, liver, and other parts of the body, and manifests itself in swelling of the legs and ankles. Increased blood pressure can be relieved by prescribing alpha blockers, which relax the smooth muscles of the arteries, prostate, and bladder neck.

- **Coronary artery disease (CAD)** affects the blood vessels that feed the heart muscle. A build up of plaque inside the vessels causes them to narrow and eventually thicken. The vessels are then unable to carry valuable blood to other parts of the body. Angina pectoris is a common form of coronary artery disease that is felt in the heart and left side of the body. This disease is relieved by taking a vasodilator, which is used to increase the diameter of the blood vessel.

The Respiratory System

Respiratory disorders are caused by infection or by the surrounding environment, especially if the body exhibits hypersensitivity to allergens in the air.

RECALL TIP

To remember which of the two types of diabetes is more likely to be fatal, use the phrase "This Is Deadly" to remember Type I Diabetes is the less common, but more deadly strain of the disease.

- **Asthma** is primarily an inflammatory disorder that affects the bronchial tubes of the lungs. Asthma is characterized by bronchospasms, airway constriction, mucous membrane swelling, and increased mucus production.

- **Emphysema** is a chronic obstructive pulmonary disorder that occurs when the alveoli are permanently enlarged due to exposure to outside irritants like cigarette smoke or air pollution.

Standard and Abnormal Laboratory Values

RECALL TIP

The abbreviation *SI* stands for Standard International Unit, which is the system of measurement used throughout most of the world. Because it is based on the metric system, its measurements are based on a factor of ten. Also, percentages are always converted to decimals. To convert a percentage to a decimal, simply move the decimal two places to the left and remove the % sign.

Diseases and disorders are often first diagnosed in a medical laboratory. This is where blood, urine, and other body samples are analyzed to identify what may be ailing the body.

Laboratory staff members take the results from these tests and compare them to normal or reference values to determine one's health. These normal laboratory values show the acceptable ranges of a healthy population. Because part of your job as a pharmacy technician will be to collect and communicate patient-specific data, it is essential to be familiar with normal laboratory test values and the numbers associated with them. It is also important to note that normal values can differ depending on the laboratory doing the testing. The table on page TK lists normal laboratory values for several common tests.

Normal Laboratory Values	
Test	**Normal Range**
Bleeding time	template: 3–6 min (SI, 3–6m); ivy: 3–6 min (SI, 3–6 m)
PTT, activated	21–35 sec (SI, 21–35 sec)
RBC Count	Men: 4.5–5.5 million/mm^3 (SI, 4.5–5.5 $\times$ 10^{12}/L) venous blood Women: 4–5 million/mm^3 (SI, 4.5–5.5 $\times$ 10^{12}/L) venous blood
WBC count	4,500–10,500 cells/mm^3
Glucose, plasma, fasting	70–110 mg/dl (SI, 3.9–6.1 mmol/L)
Glucose, plasma, 2-hour postprandial	<145 mg/dl (SI, <8 mmol/L)
Cholesterol, total serum	Men: <205 mg/dl (SI, <5.30 mmol/L) (desirable) Women: <190 mg/dl (SI, <4.90 mmol/L) (desirable)

Chapter Summary

- Your awareness of the human body's physical and structural makeup will allow you to understand how diseases can disrupt or impair the body's natural functions.

- Anatomy and physiology are closely related because form and function are intertwined. Anything that upsets the normal structure or working of the body is considered a disease.

- Epidemiology is essential for practitioners of preventative medicine to understand how health and disease affect the population as a whole.
- The difficult task of predicting when and how disease enters the body is aided by the identification of risk factors, including age, gender, heredity, living conditions, habits, emotional disturbance, physical and emotional damage, and pre-existing illness.
- Symptoms typically help doctors identify the type of disease that has entered the body. Many of these diseases affect specific body systems.
- Medical laboratory testing is an important tool for physicians in that it is used to diagnose and treat disease.
- Technicians use normal laboratory values to analyze test results to determine the health of an individual.

PRACTICE TEST QUESTIONS

Anatomy, Physiology, and Disease

1. Asthma primarily affects which part of the lungs?
   a. the alveoli
   b. the air sac
   c. the lung tissue
   d. the bronchial tubes

2. Alzheimer disease is a disorder resulting from low levels of the neurotransmitter:
   a. serotonin.
   b. dopamine.
   c. acetycholine.
   d. ephinephrine.

3. The adrenal glands are located on the:
   a. liver.
   b. kidney.
   c. thyroid.
   d. spleen.

4. The "master gland" of the endocrine system is the:
   a. adrenal gland.
   b. pineal gland.
   c. hypothalamus.
   d. pituitary gland.

5. A _____ fracture occurs during the course of normal activity due to osteoporosis.
   a. stress
   b. simple
   c. complex
   d. compound

6. The central nervous system consists of the:
   a. brain and spinal cord.
   b. brain and autonomic nervous system.
   c. spinal cord and somatic nervous system.
   d. somatic and autonomic nervous systems.

7. In emphysema, there is permanent enlargement of the:
   a. bronchi.
   b. alveoli.
   c. bronchioles.
   d. smooth muscle of the lungs.

8. Muscles that control movement such as walking or talking are controlled by the:
   a. autonomic nervous system.
   b. central nervous system.
   c. somatic nervous system.
   d. sympathetic nervous system.

9. Neurons that release the neurotransmitter norepinephrine, are referred to as:
   a. affectors.
   b. cholinergic.
   c. effectors.
   d. adrenergic.

10. The part of the brain directly involved in the control of many of the body's activities is the:
    a. cerebrum.
    b. cerebellum.
    c. hypothalamus.
    d. medulla oblongata.

11. The _____ of the peripheral nervous system are responsible for providing sensory information to the central nervous system.
    a. interneurons
    b. motor neurons
    c. efferent neurons
    d. afferent neurons

12. A relatively slow heart rate of less than 60 beats/minute is referred to as:

   a. bradycardia.
   b. tachycardia.
   c. sinus arrhythmia.
   d. congestive heart failure.

13. When calculating PTT time, the normal range runs:

   a. 5–10 sec
   b. 10–15 sec
   c. 15–20 sec
   d. 21–35

14. A patient retaining excessive fluid, resulting in swollen legs and ankles, is likely suffering from:

   a. stroke.
   b. arrhythmia.
   c. congestive heart failure.
   d. coronary artery disease.

15. Newly oxygenated blood returning from the lungs enters the heart through which chamber?

   a. left atrium
   b. right atrium
   c. left ventricle
   d. right ventricle

16. The main organ of the integumentary system is the:

   a. heart.
   b. lungs.
   c. kidneys.
   d. skin.

17. The most common risk factor associated with the development of skin cancer is:

   a. diet.
   b. smoking.
   c. sun exposure.
   d. inflammation.

18. The term *onychomycosis* is associated with:

   a. eczema.
   b. skin cancer.
   c. yeast infection.
   d. fungal infection of the nail beds.

19. Drugs prescribed to relax the smooth muscles of the arteries, the prostate, and the bladder neck to reduce blood pressure are called:

   a. vasodilators.
   b. beta blockers.
   c. alpha blockers.
   d. ACE inhibitors.

20. Angina pectoris is a coronary artery disease relieved by taking a(n):

   a. arrhythmic.
   b. vasodilator.
   c. beta blocker.
   d. calcium channel blocker.

21. Candidiasis is classified as:

   a. cancer.
   b. shingles.
   c. yeast infection.
   d. fungal infection.

22. Shingles is the reactivation of which viral infection?

   a. measles
   b. mumps
   c. influenza
   d. chicken pox

23. Hyperglycemia is seen primarily in which type of diabetes?

   a. Type I
   b. Type II
   c. gestational
   d. Insulin Resistance

24. The primary cause of Type II diabetes is:

   a. polyuria.
   b. polyphagia.
   c. ketoacidosis.
   d. insulin resistance.

25. Which adrenergic receptor is responsible for relaxing smooth muscle?

   a. beta-1
   b. alpha-1
   c. beta-2
   d. alpha-2

26. Both Alzheimer disease and Parkinsonism:

   a. involve serotonin deficiency.
   b. are curable with currently available drug therapies.
   c. are progressive in spite of currently available drug therapies.
   d. contain a defect in the enzyme that transforms tyramine to dopamine.

27. The normal range for glucose levels are:

   a. 50–70 mg
   b. 70–110 mg
   c. 150–170 mg
   d. 170–200 mg

5

Pharmacology

Test Topics

After completing this chapter, you should be able to demonstrate knowledge of the following:

1. Drug interactions (such as drug-disease, drug-drug, drug-laboratory, drug-nutrient)

2. Effects of a patient's age (for example, neonates, geriatrics) on drug and non-drug therapy

3. Drug information sources including printed and electronic reference materials

4. Pharmacology (for example, mechanism of action)

5. Common and severe side or adverse effects, allergies, and therapeutic contraindications associated with medications

6. Drug indications

7. Relative role of drug and non-drug therapy (for example, herbal remedies, lifestyle modification, smoking cessation)

Test Terms

- **additive drug reaction** when the combined effect of two drugs is equal to the sum of the separate effects of the two drugs

- **adverse effect** any undesirable effect of a drug

- **antagonistic drug reaction** when one drug interferes with another, causing the effects of one of the drugs to be lessened or completely neutralized

- **contraindications** reasons for not giving a particular drug to a patient, such as allergic reactions or preexisting conditions

- **drug indications** reasons for giving a particular drug to a patient

- **gastroesophageal reflux disease (GERD)** a condition in which the gastric contents of the stomach, including acid, back up or reflux into the esophagus

- **hyperthyroidism** a condition in which there is an increase in the amount of thyroid hormones manufactured and secreted

- **hypothyroidism** a condition in which there is a deficiency of thyroid hormone

- **pharmaceutic phase** with non-liquid oral medications, the body's dissolution of the drug so that the body can absorb it

- **pharmacokinetic phase** the process of how the body handles the drug, includes absorption, distribution, metabolism, and excretion

- **pharmacodynamic phase** the drug's effects on the body

- **pharmacology** the study of drugs and their actions on living organisms

- **synergistic drug reaction** when the combined effect of two drugs is greater than the sum of the separate effects of the two drugs

The field of pharmacology includes a broad spectrum of knowledge areas involving drugs. As a pharmacy technician student, you have learned about all of these areas, including which drugs are used to treat certain illnesses and how drugs can have undesirable effects on the body.

A health care worker who prepares and dispenses medications needs to be aware of what particular drugs do to the body and how different drugs interact with other drugs. These types of interactions can be fatal, so great care must be taken when administering drugs.

Pharmacology

Pharmacology is the study of drugs and their actions on living organisms. Those who deal with medications on a daily basis need a firm grasp of the principles of pharmacology, including knowing the different types of drugs and knowing what happens to drugs in the body.

Drugs in the Body

Once administered, drugs taken orally (except liquids) go through three phases.

- The **pharmaceutic phase** is the dissolution of the drug so that the body can absorb it.
- The **pharmacokinetic phase** refers to the process of how the body handles the drug. The processes involved in this phase are absorption (in which the drug is moved from the gastrointestinal tract to body fluids), distribution (in which the blood takes the drug to other parts of the body), metabolism (in which the liver converts the drug to inactive compounds that the body can use), and excretion (in which the excretory system removes the drug from the body).
- The **pharmacodynamic phase** is the final phase and refers to the drug's effects on the body.

Liquid medications and injections go through only the latter two phases.

> **RECALL TIP**
>
> Use the phrase "all drugs must exit" to remember the processes of the pharmacokinetic phase: absorption, distribution, metabolism, and excretion.

Drug and Non-Drug Therapy

Both drug and non-drug therapies have their place in patient treatment. Though less is understood about how non-drug therapy such as herbal therapy affects the body, many patients have found this type of therapy to be effective. In the United States, the FDA considers substances such as herbs, vitamins, and amino acids to be dietary supplements, and does not regulate them as drugs. However, vitamins can be an important part of therapy. For instance, those patients who are having trouble with blood clotting can be treated with vitamin K, a vitamin the body depends on for proper blood clotting. Patients need to keep in mind that non-drug therapy such as herbal therapy has the potential to be just as harmful as drug therapy if the herb is not used as directed or if the non-drug therapy interacts adversely with drug therapy.

> **RECALL TIP**
>
> Though the term *clotting* begins with a *c*, you can remember that vitamin K is used by the body for blood clotting if you take note of the fact that *clotting* begins with a hard *c*, which is the sound that the letter *k* makes.

Lifestyle Changes

Another form of non-drug therapy is making a lifestyle change. This can involve quitting an unhealthy habit, such as smoking, or eating more healthy foods. Some lifestyle changes are beneficial for a patient's overall health. Others are necessitated by the onset of a condition such as hypertension or anemia.

Effects of Age on Drug and Non-Drug Therapy

The age of the patient can have a great effect on both drug and non-drug therapy. Generally, the age of a patient affects the pharmacokinetic phase. The organs of infants and young children aren't as mature as those of adults, so they have a more difficult time with the metabolism and excretion of drugs. Therefore, infants and children require smaller doses. Older adult patients also react differently to drugs. An older adult patient may require a smaller dose of a drug because of decreased organ function.

Drug Indications

Drug indications refer to reasons for giving a particular drug to a patient. Proton pump inhibitors, for instance, are given to patients to treat ulcers because these drugs block acid production in the stomach. SSRIs are used to treat depression because they block the reuptake of the neurotransmitter serotonin.

One Drug, Many Indications

A certain drug can be used to treat several ailments, and clinical research can reveal new indications for a drug. For example, alpha blockers were originally used to treat hypertension but are now also used to relax smooth muscle in vascular walls. Lithium was originally used to treat gout but is now also used to treat bipolar disorder.

Drug Contraindications

In contrast to indications, **contraindications** are reasons for *not* giving a particular drug to a patient. Drugs can be contraindicated for certain patients for any number of reasons, including:

- allergic reactions
- interactions with another drug they're taking
- dietary concerns
- preexisting conditions

RECALL TIP
You can remember what a contraindication is by looking at the word part *contra*. This word part is also found in the common word *contrary*, which means "opposite" or "incompatible."

For example, because salicylates prolong bleeding time, patients who are taking anticoagulants should not also take aspirin or NSAIDs. Because beta blockers decrease the activity of the sympathetic nervous system, patients with asthma should not take these drugs. Patients taking MAOIs must maintain strict diets. A patient taking an MAOI may experience a hypertensive crisis after eating a food containing tyramine (for example, pepperoni, sour cream, yogurt, fermented cheeses, chocolate, avocados, bananas, and eggplants).

Drug Interactions

Drug interactions are important factors to consider when determining how to treat a patient. The two most important types of drug interactions are drug-drug interactions and drug-food interactions.

Drug-Drug Interactions

A drug-drug interaction occurs when a drug interacts with another drug in the body. In this type of situation, one drug may interfere with the effects of another drug. This can cause one of three types of reactions.

- An **additive drug reaction** is when the combined effect of the two drugs is equal to the sum of the separate effects of the two drugs.
- A **synergistic drug reaction** is when the combined effect of the two drugs is greater than the sum of the separate effects of the two drugs. Synergistic drug effects can be extremely dangerous.
- An **antagonistic drug reaction** is when one drug interferes with another, causing the effects of one of the drugs to be lessened or completely neutralized.

Drug-Food Interactions

Food can alter the effects of a drug, and it can also can change the rate at which the drug is absorbed by the body. Some drugs must be taken on an empty stomach so that they can be absorbed into the bloodstream more quickly. On the other hand, drugs that irritate the stomach should be taken with food to minimize the irritation. Some other drugs can combine with food to form a mixture that the body can't absorb at all. For example, a patient taking statins for high cholesterol should never eat grapefruit, as the combination of chemicals could result in a dangerous build up of the statins in the patient's system.

Drug Reactions

Drugs are administered for their therapeutic effects, which are the desired effects of the drugs. However, drugs, whether prescription or over-the-counter medications, can cause other reactions as well. These include adverse effects and allergic reactions.

Adverse Effects

Adverse effects, or side effects, can range from being mild and bearable to severe and life threatening. An **adverse effect** is any undesirable effect of a drug. For many drugs, the adverse effects are known, and it is important for you to know what the more common adverse effects are. However, some adverse effects are unpredictable and may only manifest after several doses.

Drugs can cause various types of adverse effects. For example, the most common adverse effect of antibiotics is skin rash. Tetracycline, a broad-spectrum antibiotic, commonly causes photosensitivity (abnormally heightened reactivity of the skin to sunlight). Certain components of drugs can also cause adverse effects. For example, the magnesium components of some antacids can cause diarrhea. There are other drugs that cause few adverse effects, or for which adverse effects are rare. Acetaminophen (e.g., Tylenol), a common analgesic, is relatively free of adverse effects.

The table on page TK shows the adverse effects associated with some different types of medications.

Examples of Adverse Effects of Medications		
Drug	**Drug Use**	**Adverse Effect**
acetaminophen (e.g., Tylenol)	analgesic, antipyretic	rare if used as directed; skin eruptions, urticaria, hemolytic anemia, pancytopenia, jaundice, hepatotoxicity
dopamine	shock caused by MI, trauma, open-heart surgery, renal failure	nausea, vomiting, ectopic beats, tachycardia, anginal pain, palpitations, hypotension, dyspnea

(continued)

Examples of Adverse Effects of Medications *(continued)*

Drug	Drug Use	Adverse Effect
magnesium oxide (e.g., Mag-Ox 400)	antacid	diarrhea, dehydration, nausea, vomiting, hypotension, decreased respirations
metaproterenol sulfate (Allupent)	asthma, bronchospasm	tachycardia, tremor, nervousness, shakiness, nausea, vomiting
milrinone lactate (Primacor)	heart failure	ventricular arrhythmias, hypotension, angina, chest pain, headaches, hypokalemia
norepinephrine (Levophed)	shock, hypotension, cardiac arrest	restlessness, headache, dizziness, bradycardia, hypertension
paroxetine (e.g., Paxil)	depression, OCD, anxiety disorders	headache, tremors, nervousness, dizziness, insomnia, nausea, diarrhea, visual disturbances, sweating
penicillin G (Pzizerpen)	antibiotic	rash, glossitis, stomatitis, gastritis, furry tongue, nausea, vomiting, diarrhea, fever, pain at injection site
phenobarbital	insomnia, seizures, convulsive episodes, preanesthetic	somnolence, agitation, confusion, ataxia, vertigo, CNS depression, nightmares, nausea, constipation, bradycardia, hypotension, respiratory depression
tetracycline (e.g., Sumycin)	infections caused by microorganisms	nausea, vomiting, diarrhea, hypersensitivity, photosensitivity, pseudomembranous colitis, hematologic changes, discoloration of teeth

Pharmacology Examples

The following examples of pharmacology in action demonstrate how drugs are used to treat different conditions. These examples give insight into how the various components of pharmacology come together when treating a patient.

Gastroesophageal Reflux Disease

Gastroesophageal reflux disease (GERD), also known as acid reflux, is a condition in which the gastric contents of the stomach, including acid, back up or reflux into the esophagus. This can cause damage to the lining of the esophagus. The most common symptom is this disease is heartburn. Patients who are experiencing GERD are advised to remove foods that irritate GERD from their diets, including the following:

- caffeinated beverages, such as coffee, tea, and soft drinks
- fried foods and fatty foods
- acidic foods such as citrus fruits and tomatoes

The main types of drugs used to treat GERD are antacids, gastrointestinal stimulants, H2-blockers (H2-histamine receptor antagonist drugs), and proton pump inhibitors. In the body, these drugs reduce or even eliminate acid in the stomach.

Hyperthyroidism and Hypothyroidism

A patient displaying nervousness, heat intolerance, weight loss, and a fast heart rate is most likely experiencing **hyperthyroidism**. This condition indicates an increase in the amount of thyroid hormones manufactured and secreted. Antithyroid drugs are used to treat hyperthyroidism. These drugs inhibit the manufacture and release of thyroid hormones. The body uses iodine to produce thyroid hormone, but solutions of this element can also be used to treat hyperthyroidism. Strong iodine solutions, for instance, inhibit the release of thyroid hormones. Radioactive iodine accumulates in the cells of the thyroid gland and destroys the cells.

In contrast, hypothyroidism is a condition in which there is a deficiency of thyroid hormone, which can make the patient suffer from hair loss, dry skin, sluggishness, and constipation among other symptoms. In chronic cases, hypothyroidism can lead to cretinism, a condition characterized by severely stunted growth. Thyroid hormone deficiency is generally treated with thyroid hormones and thyroid stimulating hormones.

> **RECALL TIP**
>
> To remember the difference between hyperthyroidism and hypothyroidism, just look at the prefixes. H*yper-* refers to an excess of something—in this case, thyroid hormone. *Hypo-* both rhymes with and means "low."

Drug Information Sources

There are various reference materials available that are very useful for medical professionals who prescribe and distribute medications. The following are some of the more popular references:

- The *Physicians' Desk Reference (PDR)*, updated annually, provides physicians with comprehensive information about prescription drugs. This guide includes information about dosages, contraindications, and adverse reactions for more than 3,000 drugs.
- The *Drug Topics Red Book*, also updated annually, contains essential facts and pricing information about prescription and OTC drugs, as well as medical devices and accessories. Because of its focus on arming the pharmacist with all the knowledge required to guide patients, this guide is more often found in community pharmacies than in hospital pharmacies.
- *Ident-A-Drug* comes in electronic and text versions. The database allows health care professionals to identify drugs based on the color and shape of the tables and capsules, or by the identification codes imprinted on them.
- *Facts & Comparisons*, one of the "bibles" of pharmacy, has been a source of drug information for over 50 years. It is available in many forms, including print, CD-ROM, PDA, and Internet.

Chapter Summary

- Pharmacology is the study of drugs and their effects on the body.
- Pharmacokinetics involves the processes of absorption, distribution, metabolism, and excretion.
- The age of a patient can have a great effect on the dosage that should be administered for a particular medication.
- Drugs can interact with food and with other drugs to cause unexpected effects in the body.
- Some drugs can cause adverse effects in patients. These effects can range from being mild irritations to being life threatening.
- Medical professionals have a wide variety of reference materials to choose from, including the *Physicians' Desk Reference*, the *Drug Topics Red Book*, *Ident-A-Drug*, and *Facts & Comparisons*.

PRACTICE TEST QUESTIONS

Pharmacology

1. The magnesium component of an antacid is most likely to cause:
   a. constipation.
   b. diarrhea.
   c. wheezing.
   d. rash.

2. The study of drugs and their actions on living organisms is:
   a. pharmacokinetics.
   b. pharmacodynamics.
   c. pharmaceuticals.
   d. pharmacology.

3. The class of drugs that completely shuts off acid production in the stomach is:
   a. H2 blockers.
   b. antacids.
   c. proton pump inhibitors.
   d. laxatives.

4. The most common side effect of antibiotics is:
   a. skin rash.
   b. phototoxicity.
   c. GI tract upset.
   d. hepatotoxicity.

5. A reference used more in a community pharmacy than in a hospital pharmacy is:
   a. PDR.
   b. Drug Topics Red Book.
   c. Ident-A-Drug.
   d. Facts & Comparisons.

6. Drugs have many actions. The desired action is called:
   a. side effect.
   b. physiological effect.
   c. serendipitous effect.
   d. therapeutic effect.

7. There are three phases oral drugs pass through in the body. The phase in which the drug is dissolved so the body can absorb it is called the:
   a. pharmacokinetic phase
   b. pharmacodynamic phase
   c. absorption phase
   d. pharmaceutic phase

8. Proper blood clotting is dependent on which vitamin?
   a. vitamin D
   b. vitamin K
   c. vitamin B_1
   d. vitamin A

9. Drugs originally prescribed to treat hypertension that are now being given to relax smooth muscle in vascular walls are:
   a. alpha blockers.
   b. beta blockers.
   c. thiazide diuretics.
   d. loop diuretics.

10. A reference used to identify a specific tablet or capsule by its color and shape is:
    a. PDR.
    b. Facts & Comparisons.
    c. Ident-A-Drug.
    d. Drug Topics Red Book.

11. The drug of choice to treat patients allergic to sulfa is:
    a. erythromycin.
    b. nitrofurantoin.
    c. erythromycin.
    d. metronidazole.

12. An adverse effect of a drug is considered a/an:
    a. poisoning, harmful or life threatening.
    b. anticipated and desired effect.
    c. nuisance factor.
    d. undesired effect that requires modification of treatment.

13. The process of how drugs are handled in the body is called:
    a. pharmacology.
    b. pharmacodynamics.
    c. pharmacokinetics.
    d. pharmacotherapeutics.

14. The primary site of metabolic processing is the:
    a. liver.
    b. kidney.
    c. small intestine.
    d. large intestine.

15. Patients who are taking tetracycline should avoid:
    a. iron supplements.
    b. vitamin B.
    c. zinc.
    d. sunshine.

16. The Physicians' Desk Reference (PDR) is updated:
    a. monthly.
    b. quarterly.
    c. weekly.
    d. annually.

17. Drugs go through four processes in the body. Which process converts drugs to compounds to be used by the body?

    a. absorption
    b. distribution
    c. metabolism
    d. excretion

18. The element from the diet that is used by the body to produce thyroid hormone is:

    a. sodium.
    b. aluminum.
    c. iodine.
    d. calcium.

19. A food restriction for patients taking MAOIs is:

    a. apples.
    b. fermented cheese.
    c. green leafy vegetables.
    d. beef.

20. A synergistic drug reaction is defined as:

    a. a reaction when the combined effect of the two drugs is greater than the separate effects of the two drugs.
    b. a reaction when the combined effect of the two drugs is equal to the sum of the separate effects of the two drugs.
    c. a reaction in which one drug interferes with the other, causing the effects of one of the drugs to be lessened or neutralized.
    d. none of the above.

21. A reference that is known as one of the "bibles" of pharmacy is:

    a. *PDR.*
    b. *Drug Topics Red Book.*
    c. *Ident-A-Drug.*
    d. *Facts & Comparisons.*

22. Aspirin should be prescribed with caution for patients taking:

    a. statins.
    b. beta blockers.
    c. anticoagulants.
    d. alpha blockers.

23. An analgesic that is relatively free of side effects is:

    a. meperidine.
    b. acetaminophen.
    c. morphine.
    d. hydrocodone.

24. Non-drug therapy could include such substances as:

    a. herbs
    b. vitamins.
    c. amino acids.
    d. all of the above.

25. Which of the phases that a drug passes through in the body is affected by age?

    a. pharmacokinetic phase
    b. pharmacodynamic phase
    c. pharmaceutic phase
    d. absorption phase

6

Dosage Forms, Delivery Systems, and Routes of Administration

Test Topics

After completing this chapter, you should be able to demonstrate knowledge of the following:

1. Strengths/dose, dosage forms, physical appearance, routes of administration, and duration of drug therapy
2. Delivery systems for distributing medications (for example, pneumatic tube, robotics)

Test Terms

- **buccal** drug administration in the pouch between the cheek and the gum
- **controlled-release medications** drugs designed to release at a constant, gradual rate over an extended period of time
- **elixir** drug dissolved in alcohol and flavored
- **emulsion** medication that is combined with water and oil
- **enteral medications** drugs that enter the body through the gastrointestinal tract
- **extract** a highly concentrated form of a medication, typically given in a liquid to hide its strong taste
- **Food and Drug Administration (FDA)** governing body that reviews and approves all drugs for sale in the United States
- **inert ingredients** also called pharmaceutical ingredients, non-medicinal agents delivered in combination with drug substances, e.g., preservatives
- **intramuscular (IM)** drug administration by injection into muscle
- **intravenous (IV)** drug administration directly into the blood through a vein
- **parenteral medications** drugs that do not pass through the gastrointestinal tract, e.g., injections, inhalants, and topical creams
- **subcutaneous (SubQ or SC)** drug administration by injection beneath the skin into subcutaneous tissue, usually in the patient's upper arm, thigh, or abdomen
- **sublingual (SL)** drug administration under the tongue
- **suspensions** particles of medication that are dissolved in liquid
- **syrup** sweet, flavored forms of liquid medication
- **topical** drug administration through the skin of mucous membrane

- **transdermal** drug administration of ointment, cream, or gel through the skin using a patch that releases the drug gradually
- **unit-dose system** system in which drug orders are filled and medications dispensed to fill each patient's medication order(s) for a 24-hour period

It has been said that the only difference between a drug and a poison is the dose. When a drug is developed, the most effective routes of administration must be determined. In addition, guidelines for dosage according to a variety of factors including age, weight, and degree of illness must be established. It is critically important to the health of the patient that medicines are delivered properly. The four factors that need to be considered are:

- dosage
- form
- route of administration
- duration of treatment

The life of a patient could be in your hands, and a working knowledge of drug dosage and routes of administration is necessary for keeping patients safe. It is also important to make sure patients understand the duration of their treatment. Most antibiotics, for instance, have an automatic stop date of 14 days. It is extremely important for patients to take the complete course of antibiotics, as an infection can return if antibiotics are taken improperly.

Drug Origins

Traditionally, drugs were derived from natural sources, such as:

- plants
- animals
- minerals

Today, however, laboratory researchers use traditional knowledge, along with chemical science, to develop synthetic drug sources. One advantage of chemically developed drugs is that they're free from the impurities found in natural substances. They are also more readily available, and they are less expensive to make than drugs from other sources. Synthetic drugs can be entirely man-made or semi-synthetic (composed of both natural and synthetic molecules).

Whether developed from natural or synthetic sources, drug substances are generally delivered in combination with non-medicinal agents, referred to as **inert ingredients** (or pharmaceutical ingredients). These inert ingredients do not contain the physiological effect of the drug. In addition, preservatives are sometimes added to reduce the likelihood of contamination and to increase shelf life.

> **RECALL TIP**
>
> Imagine inert ingredients as the couch potatoes of the pharmaceutical world. *Inert* means "inactive"—these ingredients don't have a therapeutic action.

Drug Approval

In the United States, all drugs must be approved by the **Food and Drug Administration (FDA)**. The drug development process, from preclinical research through clinical studies and final review by the FDA, can take from 7 to 12 years, and sometimes even longer. Even after the drug is released to the market, its safety and effectiveness continues to be monitored.

Routes of Administration

A drug's route of administration influences the rate at which the drug is absorbed and distributed in the body. These variables affect the drug's action and the patient's response. There are several different routes by which drugs can be administered.

Oral Administration

> **RECALL TIP**
>
> To remember the medical abbreviation "PO," it's helpful to know the original Latin phrase: *per os*. This phrase is translated "by mouth."

Oral (PO, or "by mouth") administration is usually the safest, most convenient, and least expensive route. For these reasons, it is the most common route of administration. This route is used only by patients who are conscious and capable of swallowing.

Bucccal and Sublingual Administration

> **RECALL TIP**
>
> To remember the meaning of the term *sublingual*, break it down into its root words. *Sub* means "under" and *lingual* refers to the tongue. Thus, sublingual medications are placed under the tongue.

Certain drugs are given **buccally** (in the pouch between the cheek and the gum) or **sublingually** (or SL, under the tongue) to prevent their destruction or transformation in the stomach or small intestine. After dissolving, these medications bypass the stomach and immediately enter the bloodstream for rapid action.

Sublingual tablets, for example, are used to treat angina attacks. When given by this route of administration, the drug is able to reach the bloodstream more quickly than if the patient had taken an oral medication.

Rectal and Vaginal Administration

Suppositories, ointments, creams, or gels may be instilled rectally (PR) or vaginally (PV) to treat local irritation or infection. Some drugs applied to the mucosa of the rectum or vagina can be absorbed systemically.

Respiratory Administration

Drugs that are available as gases or powders can be administered into the respiratory system. Drugs given by inhalation are rapidly absorbed, and medications given by devices such as the metered-dose inhaler can be self-administered.

Subcutaneous Administration

With the **subcutaneous (SubQ)** route, small amounts of a drug are injected beneath the skin and into the subcutaneous tissue, usually in the patient's upper arm, thigh, or abdomen.

Intramuscular Administration

> **RECALL TIP**
>
> Remember that *aqua* is a Latin word meaning "water." Thus, a solution that contains water is considered aqueous.

The **intramuscular (IM)** route allows drugs to be injected directly into various muscle groups at varying tissue depths. It's used to give aqueous suspensions (solutions that contain water) and solutions in oil. This route is also used to administer medications that aren't available in oral form.

Intravenous Administration

The **intravenous (IV)** route allows the injection of substances (drugs, fluids, blood or blood products, and diagnostic contrast agents) directly into the bloodstream through a vein. This is the most rapid route of administration possible. Administration can range from a single dose to an ongoing infusion delivered with great precision.

Topical Administration

The **topical** route of administration delivers a drug through the skin or a mucous membrane. Topical administration is used for most of the following preparations:

- dermatologic—creams, ointments, and gels that are applied directly to the skin
- ophthalmic—solutions that are administered to the eye, including eye drops and certain creams that are applied to the surface of the eye
- otic—solutions that are delivered into the ear
- nasal—various sprays and creams that are applied to the nasal passages

Transdermal Administration

It is increasingly common for ointments, creams, and gels to deliver drugs systemically. This is accomplished by combining the medication with various penetration enhancers. The **transdermal** patch is a useful preparation for the gradual delivery of certain medications. These patches are placed directly on the skin and are used to treat a wide variety of conditions, both local and systemic.

Dosage Forms

Proper dosage forms are needed to safely administer the appropriate dose of a drug. There are two main groupings of medications:

- enteral medications
- parenteral medications

Enteral medications enter the body through the stomach and intestines—the gastrointestinal tract. Most patients prefer to take drugs by mouth (PO), which is the easiest way to get a drug into the body. Most medicines of this kind come in a form that a patient can swallow, such as tablets, capsules, or liquids. However, some medicines cannot be given by mouth, or the body can't absorb the drug fast enough if it is taken that way. Sometimes, a patient is unconscious or not physically able to swallow a tablet or a liquid. Thus, there is another category of medications to fit these circumstances. These medications are called **parenteral medications**. They do *not* go through the gastrointestinal tract. Because these medications bypass the stomach, they deliver medication more quickly than enteral medications. Some examples of parenteral medications are injections, inhalants, and topical creams.

Solid Forms of Oral Medications

Solid forms of oral medications are often preferred, as they are the most stable, have a long shelf life, and are easy for patients to self-administer. However, one disadvantage of this dosage form is that it has a delayed onset of action. The following are several examples of solid oral dosage forms.

- A powder is a finely ground form of a medication. Some patients may find a powder hard to swallow, so most powders are stirred into a liquid.
- A capsule provides medication in powdered or granulated form that's packaged inside a gelatin casing. A capsule is designed to dissolve in stomach acids or in the small intestine.
- Tablets can be scored for patients to split into smaller portions if necessary. They usually dissolve in the gastrointestinal tract. Enteric coated tablets have dry,

compressed medication inside a coating that can resist stomach acids. An advantage of this dosage form is that its special coating allows the tablet to dissolve in the intestine. Without the coating, certain medications might be harmful to the stomach (e.g., aspirin).

- A **lozenge** is a small flavored tablet that is often used to release medication into the mouth or throat. The simplest and most common form is a cough drop.

Liquid Forms of Oral Medications

Some drugs come in liquid form, allowing for faster absorption than most solid oral medications. However, one of the disadvantages of this dosage form is that oral liquids have a shorter shelf life than solid medications. The following are several liquid forms of oral medications.

- **Syrups** are very sweet, flavored forms of a medication that are high in sugar. They are often prescribed for children.
- An **elixir** is dissolved in alcohol and flavored. This dosage form is considered a water-based solution. Prescribed mainly for adults, an elixir is less sweet than a syrup.
- An **emulsion** is a medication that is combined with water and oil, which sometimes requires multiple phases for the ingredients to mix properly. If the emulsion is completed in a single step, it is considered a single phase emulsion. Gels are an example of single phase emulsions.
- An **extract** is a highly concentrated form of a medication. It may be prescribed as drops. It's typically given in a liquid to hide its strong taste.
- **Suspensions** are particles of medication that are dissolved in liquid. Suspensions usually carry the label "Shake Well."

Controlled-Release Oral Medications

RECALL TIP

To remember the advantages of controlled-release medications, think of the acronym *ILL*:

- **I** Increased patient compliance
- **L** Less frequent dosing
- **L** Limited risk of side effects

Controlled-release medications are designed to release a drug at a constant, gradual rate over an extended period of time. Sometimes referred to as "once daily" doses, these formulations only need to be taken once in a 12- or 24-hour period, as opposed to several times a day. One advantage of this dosage form is that it allows for less frequent dosing, which helps increase patient compliance. Certain formulations, such as delayed-release tablets, are coated so they resist stomach acids and instead pass into the intestines. Another advantage is that these medications dissolve in the intestines rather than the stomach, which limits the risk of side effects.

Other Dosage Forms

Other dosage forms include:

- ointments
- creams
- gels

Drugs in these forms are intended for topical application. They may be applied to the skin, the surface of the eye, or used nasally, vaginally, or rectally. These kinds of medications are used for both local and systemic effects. An antibiotic cream is used to clear up an infection on a certain part of the body, whereas an analgesic gel patch is used to control pain in the entire body.

Creams and ointments are generally applied to the skin by hand and absorbed. Gels are often applied through the use of a transdermal patch. This is a medicated patch that is placed on the skin so the drug can be absorbed gradually. Many of the common transdermal patches are effective for 72 hours or more, which makes them convenient in terms of dosing.

Delivery Systems for Distributing Medications

A number of drug dispensing systems are used to dispense medications after they have been ordered for patients. One such system is the **unit-dose system,** in which drug orders are filled and medications dispensed to fill each patient's medication order(s) for a 24-hour period. Each dose (unit) is dispensed in a sealed package that is labeled with the drug name and dosage. Many drugs are packaged by their manufacturers in unit doses; hospital pharmacies also may prepare unit doses. This allows the pharmacy to purchase certain medications in bulk (a cost-saving measure). These medications must then be repackaged by the pharmacy in unit doses.

Technology is on the rise, with many pharmacies using computerized or automated systems to complete routine tasks. The use of robotics is also becoming more common. In many institutional settings, robotics are mainly used for unit-dose repackaging procedures, although other uses for robotics are emerging.

Another piece of modern technology that is being applied to the pharmacy is the pneumatic tube system. This is the same system that is used in a bank drive-through, which allows for objects to be sent in a plastic container through a system of tubes to a different location. The idea is that prescriptions can be packaged in a separate storage area and sent up to the pharmacy or hospital room through a pneumatic tube system. This is more prevalent in hospitals than in retail pharmacies, as medications need to be sent from a central pharmacy to various points throughout the hospital.

Chapter Summary

- Drugs are derived from natural sources, such as plants and animals, as well as from synthetic (man-made) sources. The FDA establishes guidelines for approval and use of all drugs in the United States.
- There are several different routes by which drugs can be administered. These routes include oral, buccal, sublingual, rectal, vaginal, respiratory, intravenous, intramuscular, topical, and transdermal administration.
- Drugs are manufactured in a variety of dosage forms. The two main categories are enteral medications, which enter the body through the stomach and intestines, and parenteral medications, which do *not* travel through the gastrointestinal tract.
- The pharmacy industry is changing as a result of new technologies, such as the use of robotics and pneumatic tubes in the pharmacy and hospital.
- Therapeutic agents are drugs that relieve pain and maintain health.

PRACTICE TEST QUESTIONS

Dosage Forms, Delivery Systems, and Routes of Administration

1. Buccal is a route of administration in which the medication is delivered:
   a. vaginally.
   b. by injection.
   c. inside the cheek.
   d. rectally under the tongue.

2. The most rapid route of administration for medication is:
   a. PO.
   b. SL.
   c. IV.
   d. IM.

3. Liquids that carry the direction "Shake Well" are usually:

   a. elixirs.
   b. syrups.
   c. solutions.
   d. suspensions.

4. There are several different routes of administration. The most common is:

   a. PO.
   b. SL.
   c. IV.
   d. IM.

5. Solid forms of oral medication have several advantages. One disadvantage is:

   a. longer shelf life.
   b. little or no taste.
   c. delayed onset of action.
   d. convenience of self administration.

6. Which of the following dosage forms is NOT considered topical?

   a. gel
   b. cream
   c. lozenge
   d. ointment

7. Sources of drugs include:

   a. plant sources.
   b. animal sources.
   c. synthetic sources.
   d. all of the above.

8. The agency that establishes guidelines for approval and use of all drugs in the United States is the:

   a. FDA.
   b. DEA.
   c. ATF.
   d. DFA.

9. Semi-synthetic drugs are:

   a. naturally occurring chemicals.
   b. completely artificially created.
   c. artificially created natural chemicals.
   d. composed of both natural and synthetic molecules.

10. Enteral medications enter the body through the:

    a. gastrointestinal tract.
    b. veins.
    c. rectum.
    d. nose.

11. Parenteral medications are used because:

    a. they bypass the stomach.
    b. they deliver the medication quickly.

    c. they are used by patients who are unable to take medication by mouth.
    d. all of the above.

12. Preservatives are often added to medications to:

    a. increase their shelf life.
    b. eliminate the possibility of contamination.
    c. decrease the cost if drugs are produced in larger amounts.
    d. a and b.

13. Sublingual tablets are better than solid oral medications in relieving angina attacks because:

    a. They have local effects.
    b. They are more readily available than other oral medications.
    c. They bypass the stomach entering the bloodstream for quicker relief.
    d. They are smaller than most other types of tablets and can be swallowed more easily.

14. The inert ingredients in a drug include the:

    a. flavoring.
    b. coloring.
    c. preservative.
    d. all of the above.

15. Antibiotics have an automatic stop date of:

    a. 5 days.
    b. 7 days.
    c. 10 days.
    d. 14 days.

16. There are several common uses of drugs. Therapeutic agents are drugs that:

    a. relieve pain.
    b. maintain health.
    c. assist in reaching a diagnosis.
    d. alter physiological functioning to treat a disorder.

17. One of the disadvantages of taking a liquid oral medication is:

    a. faster acting.
    b. shorter shelf life.
    c. flexibility in dosing.
    d. all of the above.

18. Robotics are mainly used in many institutional settings for:

    a. dispensing.
    b. IV admixture.
    c. inventory control.
    d. unit-dose repackaging procedures.

19. The advantage(s) of taking a controlled-release medication is:

    a. it limits the risk of side effects.
    b. it increases patient compliance.
    c. it allows for less frequent dosing.
    d. all of the above.

20. A solution containing water and ethanol is considered:

    a. soluble.
    b. aqueous.
    c. homogeneous.
    d. hydroalcoholic.

21. An elixir is a solution that is considered a(n):

    a. extract.
    b. aqueous solution.
    c. water-based solution.
    d. hydroalcoholic solution.

22. Sublingual tablets are delivered by dissolving:

    a. topically.
    b. transdermally.
    c. under the tongue.
    d. inside the cheek.

23. Enteric coated medications have an advantage because they:

    a. are tasteless.
    b. are faster acting.
    c. dissolve in the stomach.
    d. dissolve in the intestine.

24. One type of emulsion form that is considered a single phase is:

    a. gel.
    b. jelly.
    c. lotion.
    d. ointment.

25. A dosage form used to deliver medication vaginally or rectally is a(n):

    a. lotion.
    b. elixir.
    c. extract.
    d. suppository.

Pharmacy Calculations and Measurement Systems

Test Topics

After completing this chapter, you should be able to demonstrate knowledge of the following:

1. Pharmacy calculations (for example algebra, ratio and proportions, metric conversions, IV drip rates, IV admixture calculations)
2. Measurement systems (for example metric and avoirdupois)

Test Terms

- **apothecaries' system** used before the metric system was introduced; used to measure liquid volume (unit is the minim) and solid weight (unit is the grain)
- **avoirdupois system** means goods sold by weight, used for ordering and purchasing some pharmaceutical products and for weighing patients
- **body surface area (BSA)** the area covered by a person's external skin
- **dimensional analysis** method of problem solving used when two quantities are directly proportional to each other
- **drip rate** the number of drops of solution infused per minute
- **flow rate** the number of milliliters of fluids administered per hour or per minute
- **infusion time** volume to be infused divided by flow rate
- **metric system** most widely used system for measuring drugs, a decimal system based on the number 10 and multiples and subdivisions of 10
- **Percent** parts per hundred; another way to express fractions and numerical relationships
- **twenty-four-hour time** also called military time, method of keeping time by numbering the hours from 1 to 24 rather than 1 to 12 twice

To be a successful pharmacy technician, it's important to have a thorough understanding of pharmaceutical calculations. Pharmacy staff are responsible for the medications they dispense, so it's important to make sure the dosages are appropriate for each patient. Incorrect doses can be harmful and sometimes even lethal.

The core of mastering calculations involves understanding basic math calculations (such as, percentages, ratios, and proportions), different measurement systems, and conversions.

Pharmacy Calculations

To properly dispense medication, pharmacy technicians are required to be experts in the following fundamentals of calculations.

Percentages

The term *percent* means parts per hundred. Percentages are another way to express fractions and numerical relationships. Because percentages are such an important part of your work, you need to know how to convert percentages easily.

Common fractions may be converted into percentages by dividing the numerator by the denominator and multiplying by 100 (parts per hundred). For example, to change the fraction 1/4 to a percentage, you would:

1. Divide the numerator by the denominator: 1/4 = .25
2. Multiply by 100: 0.25 × 100 = 25
3. 1/4 equals 25%.

Another method you can use to change a fraction to a percentage is to divide the numerator by the denominator as described above, and then simply move the decimal point two places to the right. For example, to change 3/4 to a percentage:

1. 3 divided by 4 = 0.75
2. Move the decimal point two places to the right: 0.75 → 075.0 = 75%

In addition, you may be required to figure out the percentage of a number. For example, to answer the question "What is 15% of 300?" you would use the following steps:

1. Change the word *of* to a multiplication sign: 15% × 300
2. Convert 15% to a decimal by removing the percent sign and moving the decimal point two places to the left: 15.0% = 0.15
3. Multiply to get the answer: 0.15 × 300 = 45
4. 15% of 300 is 45.

> **RECALL TIP**
>
> A decimal and a fraction can easily be converted into a percentage using two different rules. You can remember both of them by remembering the letters DM. This can be used for fractions by remembering, **d**ivide and **m**ultiply. It can also be used for decimals by remembering, **d**ecimal point **m**ove.

Ratio and Proportion

Ratio is sometimes defined as the quotient of two like numbers. This quotient is always expressed as a fraction, and the fraction is indicating the operation of dividing the numerator by the denominator. For example, the ratio of 20 to 10 is a fraction: 20/10. The ratio is written 20:10.

A proportion is the expression of two equal ratios. It can be written in three forms.

- a:b = c:d
- a:b :: c:d
- a/b = c/d

Proportions can be used to calculate the appropriate amount of medication to dispense to each patient. In any proportion it is possible to find the value of the missing term using cross-multiplication and the equation a/b = c/d. If three of the four values are known, it is easy to calculate the value of the fourth. To do this, multiply the numerator of the first ratio (a) by the denominator of the second ratio (d). Then, multiply the numerator of the second ratio (c) by the denominator of the first ratio (b). This means that ad = cb. Finally, solve the equation to find the missing term.

For example, suppose a patient were prescribed 3900 mg of aspirin. If 3 tablets contain 975 mg, how many tablets should the patient receive?

1. First, set up the equation: 3 tablets/X tablets = 975 mg/3900mg
2. Then, find the value of the unknown variable: X = (3 × 3900)/975
3. X = 12 tablets

Dimensional Analysis

Dimensional analysis is a method of problem solving. It is an easy way to figure out drug dosages that don't require memorizing a bunch of formulas. Only one equation needs to be solved to find the answer. It can be used whenever two quantities are directly proportional to each other. This allows all the units to cancel out except for the units of the desired answer. To find the answer you're looking for, follow these six steps to answer the following problem.

A patient is ordered to receive 70 mg of enoxaparin (Lovenox). It's available in vials that contain 30mg per 0.3ml. How much should be prepared?

1. Figure out the given information: 70 mg
2. Figure out what is wanted: X ml
3. Know the equivalents you need to convert: 30mg = 0.3 ml
4. Set up your equation: (70 mg/1) × (0.3 ml/30 mg)
5. Cancel out units in that appear in both the numerator and the denominator: (70 ~~mg~~/1) × (0.3 ml/30 ~~mg~~)
6. Finally, multiply the numerators and denominators and divide the products: (70 × 0.3 ml)/(1 × 30) = 21 ml/30 = 0.7 ml

Therefore, the patient should receive 0.7 ml of Lovenox.

I.V. Drip Rates

The drip rate is the number of drops of solution that need to be infused per minute. To calculate the drip rate, you need to know the calibration for the I.V. tubing selected. Different I.V. solution sets deliver fluids at varying amounts per drop. The drop factor refers to the number of drops per milliliter of solution. The drop factor is listed on the package containing the I.V. tubing administration set. Even though pharmacy staff does not regulate I. V. fluids, pharmacy staff may be responsible for assisting medical staff to help determine the volume to be administered over a specific time.

One way to calculate the drip rate is to use the following formula:

Drip rate in drops/minute = (total milliliters/total minutes) × drop factor in drops/ml

For example, suppose a patient needs an infusion of dextrose 5% in water (D_5W) at 125ml/hour. If the tubing set is calibrated at 15 gtt/ml, what is the drip rate?

1. First, convert 1 hour to 60 minutes to fit the formula.
2. Then set up the equation: X = (125 ml /60 minutes) × (15 gtt/ml)
3. Cancel out the units that appear in the numerator and the denominator:
4. X = (125 ~~ml~~ /60 minutes) × (15 gtt/~~ml~~)
5. Solve for X by dividing the numerator by the denominator: X = (125 × 15 gtt)/60 minutes
6. X = 31.25 gtt/minutes
7. The drip rate is 31.25 gtt/min.

Flow Rate

The flow rate is the number of milliliters of fluids to administer over 1 hour (or per minute). To figure out the flow rate, you need to know the total volume to be infused in milliliters and the amount of time for the infusion. Use the following formula:

RECALL TIP

To remember how to calculate the flow rate, think about how fast you flow down the street. When you drive, walk, or ride a bike, you can calculate your pace as miles per hour. The flow rate is similar except instead of miles per hour, you are figuring out volume per hour.

Flow rate = (total volume ordered/number of hours)

For example, suppose a patient needs 250 ml of normal saline solution over two hours. What is the flow rate?

- X = (250 ml/2 hours) = 125
- The flow rate is 125 ml/hr.

Infusion Time

Once you figure out the drip rate and the flow rate, you can compute the time required to infuse a specified volume of I.V. fluid. This calculation will help keep the infusion on schedule. To calculate the infusion time, you need to know the flow rate in milliliters per hour and the volume to be infused. Here's the formula:

Infusion time = (volume to be infused/flow rate)

Let's use the formula to calculate the flow rate for a sample problem. Suppose a patient requires 1 L of D_5W at 50 ml/hr. What is the infusion time?

1. First, convert 1 L to 1000 ml to make the units equivalent.
2. Then, set up the equation:
3. X = (1000 ml)/(50 ml/hr)
4. Cancel out the units that appear in the numerator and the denominator:
5. X = (1000 ~~ml~~)/(50 ~~ml~~/hr)
6. Solve for X by dividing the numerator by the denominator: X = 20 hours
7. The D_5W will infuse in 20 hours.

Body Surface Area

A person's body surface area (BSA) is the area covered by a person's external skin. It is calculated in square meters (m^2) according to height and weight. The BSA is used to calculate safe pediatric dosages for all drugs and safe dosages for adult patients receiving extremely potent drugs or drugs requiring great precision. Use the following formula to calculate a person's BSA using centimeters (cm) and kilograms (kg):

Body surface area in m^2 = $\sqrt{[(\text{height in cm} \times \text{weight in kg})/3{,}600]}$.

You can also use a modified version of the formula to calculate a person's BSA using inches (in) and pounds (lb), as shown:

Body surface area in m^2 = $\sqrt{[(\text{height in in} \times \text{weight in lb})/3{,}131]}$.

Let's use the formula to calculate the BSA for a sample problem. Calculate the BSA for a child whose weight is 27.3 kg and height is 59.5 cm.

1. $\sqrt{[(59.5 \text{ cm} \times 27.3)/3600]}$
2. $\sqrt{(1624.35/3600)}$
3. $\sqrt{.45}$
4. .67
5. The BSA for the child is .67 m^2

Calculating Dosages Using Body Surface Area

The following formula is used to calculate pediatric dosages based on a patient's BSA:

Dosage in mg = BSA $\times$ [(pediatric dose in mg)/(m^2/day)]

For example, a doctor orders ephedrine 100 mg/m²/day for a child with a BSA of 0.96 m². How much ephedrine should the child take daily?

1. $X = 0.96 \text{ m}^2 \times [(100 \text{ mg})/(1 \text{ m}^2/\text{day})]$
2. $X = 0.96 \; \cancel{\text{m}^2} \times [(100 \text{ mg})/(1 \; \cancel{\text{m}^2}/\text{day})]$
3. $X = 0.96 \times (100 \text{ mg/day})$
4. $X = 96 \text{ mg/day}$
5. The child needs 96 mg of ephedrine per day.

Measurement Systems

Medication is primarily prepared using the metric system. However, knowledge of the apothecaries', avoirdupois, household, and time systems are still required.

Metric System

The metric system is the most widely used system for measuring drugs. It is a decimal system that is based on the number 10 and multiples and subdivisions of 10. The basic units of measurement for the metric system are meters (m) for length, liters (L) for volume, and grams (g) for weight.

Equivalences of Common Metric Measurements	
1,000 mm	100 cm
100 cm	1 m
1,000 mL	1 L
10 cc	1 mL
1,000 mcg	1 mg
1,000 mg	1 g
1,000 g	1 kg

RECALL TIP

To help remember how to convert denominations within the metric system, think about the letters *R* and *L*. To reduce the denomination, move the decimal point to the right. To make the denomination larger, move the decimal point to the left.

Because the metric system is based on the decimal system, conversion within the metric system can be done by simply moving the decimal point. To change a metric denomination to the next smaller denomination, move the decimal point one place to the right. To change a metric denomination to the next larger denomination, move the decimal point one place to the left.

In pharmacy and healthcare in general, common units of measure differ by 1000. Micrograms, milligrams, grams, and kilograms are metric units of weight, and milliliters and liters measure volume. Therefore, conversions for these units can be made by moving the decimal point three places to the right to convert from larger to smaller units and three places to the left to convert smaller to larger units.

The Apothecaries' System

Doctors and pharmacists used the apothecaries' system before the metric system was introduced. Even though the apothecaries' system is rarely seen anymore, it is important to be familiar with it.

Converting from Larger to Smaller, Moving Three Places to the Right

Larger	Smaller
1.23355 kg	1,233.55 g
1,233.55 g	1,233,550 mg
1,233,550 mg	1,233,550,000 mcg
Therefore, 1.23355 kg = 1,233.55 g = 1,233,550 mg = 1,233,550,000 mcg	

Converting from Smaller to Larger, Moving Three Places to the Left

Smaller	Larger
9,876,160 mcg	9876.16 mg
9876.16 mg	9.87616 g
Therefore, 9,876,160 mcg = 9876.16 mg = 9.87616 g	

The apothecaries' system is only used to measure liquid volume and solid weight. The basic unit of measure for volume is the minim, and the basic unit of measure for weight is the grain. A minim is approximately the size of a drop of water, which is also weighs about the same as a grain of wheat. Thus, 1 drop = 1 minim = 1 grain.

Apothecaries' System Basics

Liquid Volume	
60 minims (m)	1 fluidram
8 fluidrams	1 fluid ounce (oz)
16 fluid oz	1 pint (pt)
2 pt	1 quart (qt)
Solid Weight	
60 grains (gr)	1 dram
8 drams	1 oz
12 oz	1 pound (lb)

Avoirdupois System

The avoirdupois system, which means goods sold by weight, is used for ordering and purchasing some pharmaceutical products and for weighing patients. The solid units of weight include grains (gr), ounces (oz), and pounds (lb). One ounce equals 480 gr, and 1 lb equals 16 oz or 7,680 gr. Note that the apothecaries' pound equals 12 oz, but the avoirdupois pound equals 16 oz.

The Household System

The household system of measure is the least accurate of all the systems because of the inaccuracy of the measuring devices used. However, this is the system that is used most commonly to give directions to patients.

Common Household Abbreviations and Equivalents		
Abbreviation	**Unit**	**Equivalent**
gtt	Drop	n/a
tsp	Teaspoon	n/a
tbs	Tablespoon	1 tbs = 3 tsp
oz	Fluidounce	2 tbs = 1 oz
oz	Ounce (weight)	16 oz = 1 lb
cup	Cup	1 cup = 8 oz
pt	Pint	1 pint = 2 cups
qt	Quart	1 quart = 4 cups = 2 pt

RECALL TIP

To remember which measurements are part of the household system, think about measurements you use at home. Whenever you bake or need to give yourself a dose of medicine, you'll use teaspoons, tablespoons, or cups.

Measurement of Time

Twenty-four-hour time is a method of keeping time by numbering the hours from 1 to 24 rather than 1 to 12 twice. Hour 1 begins at midnight, and hour 13 begins at 1 PM. The system uses 4 digits and no colon; therefore, 9 PM is given as 2100. The first two digits represent the hour, and the last two digits represent the minutes.

The health care system commonly uses 24-hour time to avoid giving doses at the wrong time because AM and PM were poorly written on orders. The 24-hour clock is also known as military or international time.

Conversions

Pharmacy technicians must master conversions in the metric system.

Conversions Between Systems of Measurement

The household system is commonly used on prescription labels, and therefore conversions between the metric system and the household system must be memorized. Other equivalent measures that require memorization include specific apothecary and avoirdupois measures. The following tables represent common measurements. Items in bold must be committed to memory.

Conversion Equivalents of Volume

Apothecary Measure	Approximate Metric Equivalent (mL)	Exact Metric Equivalent (mL)
1 fl oz	30	29.57
4 fl oz	120	118.28
1 pt (16 fl oz)	480	473.00
1 qt (2 pt)	960	946.00
1 gal (4 qt)	3,840	3,785.00

Conversion Equivalents of Weight

Apothecary or Avoirdupois Measure	Approximate Metric Equivalent	Exact Metric Equivalent
1 avoir oz	30 g	28.35 g
1 avoir lb (16 oz)	n/a	454 g
2.2 avoir lb	1 kg	1,000 g

Common Household Measures

Household Measure	Approximate Equivalent	Apothecary Equivalent	Other Equivalent
½ tsp	2.5 mL	n/a	n/a
1 tsp	5 mL	1 fluidram	n/a
3 tsp	15 mL	n/a	1 tbs or ½ oz
2 tbs	30 mL	1 fl oz	1 oz

Temperature Conversion

To convert Fahrenheit to Celsius, subtract 32 from the temperature in Fahrenheit and then divide by 1.8. The formula is expressed this way:

$$C = (F - 32)/1.8$$

For example, to convert 98° Fahrenheit to Celsius, you would use the following steps:

1. $98 - 32 = 66$
2. $66 \div 1.8 = 36.7$
3. 98° Fahrenheit equals 36.7° Celsius.

To convert Celsius to Fahrenheit, multiply the temperature in Celsius by 1.8 and then add 32. Here is the formula:

$$F = (C \times 1.8) + 32$$

For example, to convert 36° Celsius to Fahrenheit, you would do the following:

1. $36 \times 1.8 = 64.8$
2. $64.8 + 32 = 96.8$
3. 36° Celsius equals 96.8° Fahrenheit

Weight Conversion

To convert a patient's weight from pounds to kilograms, divide the number of pounds by 2.2. To convert a patient's weight from kilograms to pounds, multiply the number of kilograms by 2.2.

For example, to convert 50 pounds to kilograms, you would follow these steps:

1. $50 \div 2.2 = 22.7$
2. 50 pounds equals 22.7 kg.

Chapter Summary

- Pharmacists and pharmacy technicians should be experts in the fundamentals of calculations.
- Percentages are another way to express fractions and numerical relationships.
- Common fractions can be converted into percents by dividing the numerator by the denominator and multiplying by 100.
- A ratio is the quotient of two like numbers.
- A proportion is the expression of two equal ratios.
- In any proportion it is possible to find the value of the missing term using cross multiplication.
- Dimensional analysis is a method of problem solving that involved placing all of the arithmetical terms involved into one equation.
- The drip rate is the number of drops of solution that need to be infused per minute. To calculate the drip rate, you need to know the calibration for the I.V. tubing selected.

  Drip rate in drops/minute = (total milliliters/total minutes) X drop factor in drops/ml

- The flow rate is the number of milliliters of fluids to administer over 1 hour (or per minute).

  Flow rate = (total volume ordered/number of hours)

- Once you figure out the drip rate and the flow rate, you can compute the time required for infusion of a specified volume of I.V. fluid.

  Infusion time = (volume to be infused/flow rate)

- A person's body surface area (BSA) is the area covered by a person's external skin.

  Body surface area in m^2 = $\sqrt{[(\text{height in cm} \times \text{weight in kg})/3,600]}$

- The BSA allows health care workers to calculate pediatric doses.

  Dosage in mg = BSA $\times$ [(pediatric dose in mg)/(m^2/day)]

- The metric system is a decimal system that is based on the number 10 and multiples and subdivisions of 10. The basic units of measurement for the metric system are meters (m) for length, liters (L) for volume, and grams (g) for weight.

- The apothecary system is only used to measure liquid volume and solid weight. The basic unit of measure for volume is the minim, and the basic unit of measure for weight is the grain.

- The avoirdupois system is used for ordering and purchasing some pharmaceutical products and for weighing patients.

- The household system is the least accurate of all the systems and is used most commonly to give directions to patients.

- 24-hour time is a method of keeping time by numbering the hours from 1 to 24 rather than 1 to 12 twice.

- Pharmaceutical technicians must master conversions in the metric system.

- To convert Fahrenheit to Celsius, subtract 32 from the temperature in Fahrenheit and then divide by 1.8. To convert Celsius to Fahrenheit, multiply the temperature in Celsius by 1.8 and then add 32.

- To convert a patient's weight in pounds to kilograms, divide the number of pounds by 2.2. To convert a patient's weight in kilograms to pounds, multiply the number of kilograms by 2.2.

PRACTICE TEST QUESTIONS

Pharmacy Calculations and Measurement Systems

1. How many grams of drug in is a 500 mL IV bag labeled 5% Dextrose in water?
   a. 5 g
   b. 15 g
   c. 25 g
   d. 50 g

2. How many grams are in 1700 mg?
   a. 17 g
   b. 1.7 g
   c. 1,700,000 g
   d. 0.17 g

3. Calculate the dosage and mL/hr flow rate for the following drug. Propofol 5 mcg/kg/min is ordered for an 80.3 kg patient. The solution strength is 1 g/100 mL D5W.
   a. 5 mL/hr
   b. 10 mL/hr
   c. 40 mL/hr
   d. 2 mL/hr

4. Calculate the flow rate in gtt/min for an IV infusing 100 mL/hour using a 10 gtt/mL set. The resulting flow rate is:
   a. 60 gtt/min
   b. 17 gtt/min
   c. 20 gtt/min
   d. 4 gtt/min

5. Determine the BSA for a child whose weight is 35.9 kg and height is 63.5 cm.
   a. 0.80 m^2
   b. 0.85 m^2
   c. 1.50 m^2
   d. 1.16 m^2

6. Convert 75° Celsius to Fahrenheit.
   a. 157° F
   b. 164° F
   c. 167° F
   d. 183° F

7. Convert 33.2 kg to pounds.
   a. 15 lb
   b. 17 lb
   c. 33 lb
   d. 73 lb

8. Convert 45 mL to tablespoon(s).
   a. 2 tbs
   b. 3 tbs
   c. 9 tbs
   d. 12 tbs

9. Convert 35° Fahrenheit to Celsius.
   a. 2° C
   b. 6° C
   c. 4° C
   d. 10° C

10. Calculate the completion time for the following infusion. An IV with a restart time of 9:07 p.m. has an infusion time of 6 hr 27 min.

    a. 3:34 p.m.
    b. 12:37 p.m.
    c. 3:34 a.m.
    d. 2:34 p.m.

11. Convert 90 mL to ounces.

    a. 27 oz
    b. 30 oz
    c. 15 oz
    d. 3 oz

12. Change 5:15 to a percentage.

    a. 3%
    b. 33.3%
    c. 39%
    d. 45%

13. How many mcg are in 65 mg?

    a. 65,000 mcg
    b. 0.065 mcg
    c. 0.65 mcg
    d. 6500 mcg

14. Determine a child's dosage with a BSA of 0.81 m^2 receiving a drug with a recommended dosage of 40 mg/m^2.

    a. 30 mg
    b. 35 mg
    c. 32 mg
    d. 33 mg

15. Your stock solution contains 10 mg of active ingredient per 5 mL of carrier vehicle. The physician has ordered a dose of 4 mg. How many mL of stock solution will have to be administered?

    a. 2 mL
    b. 4 mL
    c. 6 mL
    d. 8 mL

16. What is 20% of 60?

    a. 6
    b. 12
    c. 10
    d. 3

17. Your pharmacy has Demerol 100 mg/mL syringes on hand. You receive an order for Demerol 75 mg IM prn pain. How many mL will the nurse give?

    a. 1 mL
    b. 0.2 mL
    c. 0.5 mL
    d. 0.8 mL

18. A suspension of naladixic acid contains 250 mg/5 mL. The syringe contains 15 mL. What is the dose (in milligrams) contained in the syringe?

    a. 750 mg
    b. 500 mg
    c. 725 mg
    d. 250 mg

19. How many 2 tsp doses can a patient take from a bottle containing 3 fl oz?

    a. 10 doses
    b. 5 doses
    c. 9 doses
    d. 12 doses

20. Find the missing term in the ratio. 1:4::x:8

    a. 4
    b. 5
    c. 6
    d. 2

21. Calculate the dosage and mL/hr flow rate for Nipride 3 mcg/kg/min has been ordered for an 87.4 kg patient. The solution has a strength of 50 mg, Nipride in 250 mL D5W.

    a. 79 mL/hr
    b. 78 mL/hr
    c. 80 mL/hr
    d. 77 mL/hr

22. A 10% solution of 200 mL contains how many grams of drug?

    a. 10 g
    b. 15 g
    c. 20 g
    d. 2 g

23. An I.V. additive has a dosage available of 30 mEq/20 mL. A dosage of 15 mEq has been ordered. How many mL will you give?

    a. 5 mL
    b. 7 mL
    c. 10 mL
    d. 15 mL

24. Determine the BSA for an adult whose weight is 175 lb and height is 67 inches.

    a. 1.80 m^2
    b. 1.81 m^2
    c. 1.93 m^2
    d. 1.94 m^2

25. A critical care patient has orders for a continuous morphine drip. The order is for 25 mg/50 mL to infuse at 8 mg/hr. Calculate the mL/hr flow rate.

    a. 8 mL/hr
    b. 16 mL/hr

c. 5 mL/hr
d. 6 mL/hr

26. Convert 3500 mg to grams
    a. 0.35 g
    b. 35 g
    c. 3.5 g
    d. 350 g

27. The doctor ordered 0.015 g of Inderal. How many milligrams is the pharmacy technician going to dispense?
    a. 1.5 mg
    b. 0.15 mg
    c. 150 mg
    d. 15 mg

28. Convert 20° Fahrenheit to Celsius
    a. 7°C
    b. 17°C
    c. −7°C
    d. −17°C

29. The pharmacy technician is asked to prepare a 3% ointment of 45 grams. The stock on hand is 10% ointment and 1% ointment. What is the final weight of the 10% ointment?
    a. 10 g
    b. 100 g
    c. 5 g
    d. 15 g

30. Change the 2:5 to a percentage
    a. 20%
    b. 250%
    c. 40%
    d. 15%

31. Change the ratio 21:35 into a fraction
    a. 3/4
    b. 1/5
    c. 1/4
    d. 3/5

32. Convert 120 mL to ounces.
    a. 4 oz
    b. 24 oz
    c. 12 oz
    d. 15 oz

33. The pharmacy receives an order for a 30 day supply of Lasix 10 mg to be given four times a day. How many tablets must the technician prepare?
    a. 50 tablets
    b. 100 tablets
    c. 120 tablets
    d. 90 tablets

34. How many milliliters is in 20 liters?
    a. 2000 mL
    b. 20,000 mL
    c. 200 mL
    d. 200,000 mL

35. An IV of 200 mL of 10% Dextrose was discontinued after only 150 mL had been infused. How many grams of dextrose was delivered?
    a. 5 g
    b. 50 g
    c. 25 g
    d. 15 g

36. Convert 24 pounds to kilograms
    a. 11.2 kg
    b. 10.9 kg
    c. 12.4 kg
    d. 52.8 kg

37. Determine the body surface area of a child who weighs 35.9 kg and 63.5 cm in height.
    a. 0.63 m²
    b. 0.61 m²
    c. 0.8 m²
    d. 0.82 m²

38. An adult is to receive a drug with a recommend dosage of 10−20 units per m². The BSA is 1.93 m². What is the recommended range for this patient?
    a. 19−39 units
    b. 20−38 units
    c. 9−18 units
    d. 18−38 units

39. How much sodium chloride is in 250 mL of D5NS?
    a. 22.5 g
    b. 2.5 g
    c. 2 g
    d. 12.5 g

40. Divide 700 by 1800 and express the answer to the nearest tenth.
    a. 0.38
    b. 0.39
    c. 0.4
    d. 0.3

41. How many micrograms are in 30 milligrams?
    a. 300 mcg
    b. 0.03 mcg
    c. 0.3 mcg
    d. 30,000 mcg

42. A dosage of 0.2 g has been ordered. The strength available is 0.5 g/5 mL. How many milliliters needs to be prepared?
    a. 2 mL
    b. 2.5 mL
    c. 3 mL
    d. 4 mL

43. Convert a child weighing 25.3 kg to pounds.
    a. 55 lb
    b. 50 lb
    c. 54 lb
    d. 56 lb

44. Calculate the BSA of a man weighting 108 kg and whose height is 194 cm.
    a. 5.82 m²
    b. 58.2 m²
    c. 2.41 m²
    d. 24.1 m²

45. The pharmacy receives an order for 1.5 g of Pencillin G to be given by IM. The stock vial contains 500 mg/1 mL. How many milliliters need to be dispensed?
    a. 3 mL
    b. 5 mL
    c. 10 mL
    d. 15 mL

46. Convert the weight of a 125 lb adult to kilograms.
    a. 52.7 kg
    b. 55.4 kg
    c. 56.8 kg
    d. 57.2 kg

47. Calculate the BSA for an adult weighting 165 lb and is 67" in height.
    a. 1.87 m²
    b. 1.88 m²
    c. 1.89 m²
    d. 1.92 m²

48. An IV medication of 25 mL is order to infuse in 30 min. The set calibration is 60 gtt/mL. Calculate the gtt/min flow rate.
    a. 15 gtt/min
    b. 20 gtt/min
    c. 30 gtt/min
    d. 50 gtt/min

49. Convert 30 mL to teaspoon(s).
    a. 2 tsp
    b. 4 tsp
    c. 6 tsp
    d. 8 tsp

50. The pharmacy technician is asked to prepare an injection of Thorazine® 30mg from a stock vial of 25mg/mL. How many milliliters will the technician draw up?
    a. 0.5 mL
    b. 1.1 mL
    c. 1.2 mL
    d. 1.5 mL

51. How would 8:30 PM be expressed in 24-hour time?
    a. 21:30
    b. 2200
    c. 2130
    d. 22:00

Sterile Products and Pharmacy Equipment

Test Topics

After completing this chapter, you should be able to demonstrate knowledge of the following:

1. Techniques, equipment, and supplies for drug administration
2. Monitoring and screening equipment
3. Medical and surgical appliances and devices
4. Automated dispensing technology
5. Procedures to prepare IV admixtures
6. Procedures to prepare chemotherapy
7. Procedures to prepare total parenteral nutrition (TPN) solutions
8. Procedures to prepare reconstituted injectable and non-injectable medications
9. Specialized procedures to prepare injectable medications
10. Procedures to prepare radiopharmaceuticals
11. Procedures to compound sterile non-injectable products
12. Aseptic techniques

Test Terms

- **area of turbulence** a triangular-shaped area in front of the beaker in which is a mixture of HEPA air and unfiltered room air
- **biological safety cabinet (BSC)** a type of hood that blows HEPA-filtered air vertically downward through a top hood and into grills located along the front and back edges of the work surface area and that has a clear glass or plastic shield
- **catheter** a delivery or drainage tube that is inserted into a vein, artery, or body cavity
- **clean room** an area in which the air quality, temperature, and humidity are highly regulated to reduce the risk of cross-contamination
- **contaminant** any unwanted particulate matter or sickness-inducing agent
- **critical area** a place where CSPs, containers, and closures are exposed to the environment
- **critical site** location where contaminants might come into contact with a CSP
- **compound sterile product (CSP)** a mixture of one or more substances that is made sterile, or free of contamination, before use
- **HEPA** filtered high-efficiency particulate air
- **infusion pump** an automatic device used with an IV system for delivering medication at regular intervals in specific quantities
- **intravenous (IV) injection** an injection directly into a vein
- **intravenous push (IVP)** a small volume of medicine injected into a vein and administered over a short period of time
- **intravenous piggybacks (IVPB)** administered on a set schedule, smaller IV bags that are added on, or "piggybacked," to a large-volume IV bag
- **laminar airflow hood (LAH)** a work area that prefilters large contaminants from the workspace and then uses

HEPA-filtered air in a horizontal flow to extract smaller particles

- **large-volume IV bag** often used for fluid replacement or for maintenance of fluids, administered continually
- **multiple-dose vials** vials that allow access to the contents of the vial more than once
- **parenterals** CSPs that are injected
- **single-dose vials** contain one dose of medication and are discarded after one use
- **sterile** free from contaminants
- **sterilization** the destruction and removal of all living organisms and their spores from a preparation
- **total nutrition admixture (TNA)** also known as total parenteral nutrition, IV therapy that provides nutrition to patients who cannot take nourishment by mouth
- **total parenteral nutrition (TPN)** also known as total nutrition admixture, IV therapy that provides nutrition to patients who cannot take nourishment by mouth

In the past, pharmacists were traditionally required to compound anything the physician ordered. Today, as a pharmacy technician, you may encounter many medications that will come from the manufacturer already prepared. However, there is a wide range of products that simply cannot be prepared ahead of time or outside of a sterile setting. To prepare these orders, the pharmacy staff must understand the processes of sterile compounding.

The Importance of Sterility

One of your most important tasks as a pharmacy technician is preparing compound sterile products, also known as CSPs. A **CSP** is a mixture of one or more substances that is made sterile, or free of contamination, before use. As you might guess, a CSP must be sterile before it comes into contact with living tissue. If the product is contaminated, the results could be lethal.

Basic Product Sterility

The term **sterilization** refers to the destruction and removal of all living organisms and their spores from a preparation. There are five basic methods used to sterilize pharmaceutical products:

- steam
- dry heat
- filtration
- gas
- ionizing radiation

Clean Room

To prepare sterile products, you must start with a sterile environment. This environment is referred to as a clean room. A **clean room** is an area in which the air quality, temperature, and humidity are highly regulated to reduce the risk of cross-contamination. Some of the initial requirements for a clean room include:

- air quality that meets the International Organization for Standardization (ISO) class standards
- filtered high-efficiency particulate air (or **HEPA**)
- access that is available only to those personnel who are trained and authorized to perform sterile compounding and facility cleaning

Contaminants

Once a CSP is prepared, it must remain **sterile**, or free from contaminants. A **contaminant** is any unwanted particulate matter or sickness-inducing agent. The most likely way for contamination to occur is by touch contamination. This happens when physical contact between a CSP and another object results in contamination of the CSP. Any time you handle a CSP, there is a risk of touch contamination. Tiny fibers are constantly falling from your clothes, your hair, and your skin. This is why it is especially important that you wear protective clothing and gloves when handling a CSP. Protective clothing and garb that covers the hair and does not shed fibers lowers the risk of touch contamination. You should also make sure that you use appropriate hand-washing techniques when required.

Critical Site

A **critical site** is any location where contaminants might come into contact with a CSP. This could be any opening or surface on which CSPs and contaminants can meet. Remember that CSPs can also come in contact with contaminants from the air. Some critical sites are frequently exposed to the air and any contaminants it contains. These include:

- the tip of a sterile syringe
- the plunger of a syringe
- the opened ampule of a drug
- an injection port

RECALL TIP

To help you remember the difference between a critical site and a critical area, remember that a critical site is a very specific place, such as the tip of a syringe. A critical area is just like it sounds, a general area, such as a laminar airflow workbench.

Critical Area

The terms *critical site* and *critical area* sound similar and mean similar things. You already know what a critical site is. A **critical area** is a place where CSPs, containers, and closures are exposed to the environment. This is where sterile products can be safely prepared or compounded while keeping the risk of contamination very low. A laminar airflow workbench or hood is an acceptable critical area.

High-Efficiency Particulate Air Filtration

In order to satisfy the U.S. Pharmacopeia's guidelines for Class 100 environments, high-efficiency particulate air filters, or HEPA filters, are used in all aseptic processing areas. The class number of an environment is used to describe the air quality in that designated area. The class numbers, such as 100 or 10,000, refer to the number of particles in the air. A Class 100 environment is the minimum area classification for preparing sterile compounds. HEPA filters are certified to provide air that is filtered with minimum 0.3-micron particle-retaining efficiency of 99.97%.

Laminar Airflow Workbench

Most CSPs are compounded in a laminar airflow workbench, also known as a **laminar airflow hood (LAH)**. The LAH is a work area that prefilters large contaminants from the workspace and then uses HEPA-filtered air in a horizontal flow to extract smaller particles. The air within the preparation space is constantly circulated away from the pharmacy technician and into an area called the airflow hood. Within the hood, the air is filtered and vented directly to the outside. In this way, the contaminants and fumes are kept in the hood of the work area—away from the product and from you. When using a horizontal airflow hood, be sure to work a minimum of 6 inches inside the front edge of the hood to help prevent contamination from the room air.

This process creates an aseptic work area.

Area of Turbulence

Remember that in most "hooded" work areas, the HEPA (filtered) air is moving horizontally. This means the air is being blown toward you in a straight line. A hooded area with no objects inside contains only HEPA filtered air. So what happens once you introduce an object into the hood? As part of your job, you will need to move objects like beakers and vials, and even your own hands, into the hood. This creates an area where HEPA air mixes with unfiltered room air.

Consider this example. When you set a beaker inside a laminar hood, filtered air moves toward the beaker in a straight line. When this air reaches the beaker, it has to move around it. This creates a triangular-shaped area in front of the beaker. In this area is a mixture of HEPA air and unfiltered room air. This area is also referred to as the **area of turbulence**.

As the beaker increases in size, so does the area of turbulence. Always place objects in a straight line, side by side, when setting them inside a hooded area. Never place them in front or in back of each other.

Biological Safety Cabinet

Unlike the LAHF described above, some hoods blow HEPA-filtered air vertically downward through a top hood and into grills located along the front and back edges of the work surface area. This kind of vertical flow hood is known as a **biological safety cabinet (BSC)**.

BSCs also have a clear glass or plastic shield that extends partially down the front of the hood. This shield and the vertical flow of air protect you from contamination by any drugs processed within.

Hazardous Drugs

Both types of hoods can be used for most product preparations, but you're required to use a BSC when working with hazardous compounds such as products used in chemotherapy treatment or cytotoxic drugs. Use aseptic techniques in all procedures for preparing these sterile products. Remove jewelry and wash hands and forearms with germicidal soap. Put on a clean, low-shedding gown and hair and foot covers. For these drugs, double-glove and use a facemask. To assure sterility, wipe down the biological safety cabinet surfaces with 70% Isopropyl Alcohol using sterile 4×4's. Assemble necessary materials. Wipe diaphrames of vials and IV ports with alcohol swabs.

Compounding Aseptic Isolator

A compounding aseptic isolator is a LAH that is completely enclosed. You can only access the work surface through glove box-type openings. Materials and supplies for aseptic processing enter through special air-lock boxes attached to the unit.

Delivery Systems

As you know, pharmacy technicians prepare many different sterile compounds. Each of these compounds is designed to use a specific route of administration in order to be effective. The pieces of equipment that cause a drug to follow its designated route of administration are referred to as the drug's delivery system.

Syringes

One of the most familiar pieces of delivery system equipment is the medical syringe. Syringes are made of glass, plastic, or metal. They are used for:

- injection
- irrigation
- withdrawal of fluids
- other parenteral delivery

Types of Syringes

Syringes vary in size from 1 mL (or 1 cc) to 60 mL (or 60 cc). The 3-mL hypodermic syringe is the most commonly used.

All hypodermic syringes are marked with calibrations showing divisions of milliliters or smaller, depending on the size of the syringe. The other side of the syringe may be marked in minims (m), a very small fluid measure equivalent to about a drop.

Two special types of syringes used to administer medications are tuberculin syringes and insulin syringes.

Tuberculin Syringe Tuberculin (TB) syringes are narrow and have a total capacity of 1 mL. Each TB syringe has 100 calibration lines. TB syringes are used for:

- newborn doses
- pediatric doses
- intradermal skin tests
- small doses in adults
- injections just beneath the skin

Insulin Syringe Insulin syringes are used only for administering insulin to diabetic patients. The insulin syringe has a total capacity of 1 mL, but uses a different calibration system than other syringes.

The 1-mL volume is marked in units (U). The units represent the strength of the insulin per milliliter. Most of the insulin that is used today is U-100, which means that it has 100 units of insulin per milliliter. On the syringe, large lines mark each group of ten units. Five smaller lines divide the ten units into groups of two. Each small line represents two units.

Syringe Sterility

When working with syringes, you must open the syringe package within the air space of the laminar airflow hood in order to preserve its sterility.

Most syringes are manufactured with a needle and cap or a protective covering over the tip. If the syringe is packaged with just a protective covering, you must not remove the covering until a needle is ready to be attached. You should complete this process as quickly as possible to avoid contamination. In addition, don't use a needle that does not have the packaging intact. It may be contaminated.

Gauge of a Needle

The gauge of a needle refers to the diameter of the opening, or lumen. Needle gauges usually range from 30 to 16. However, the *larger* the gauge, the *smaller* the opening of the needle will be. A 30-g needle, for example, has a much smaller opening than an 18-g needle.

RECALL TIP

To help remember how gauge relates to a needle, remember that a gauge and a needle have an *inverse* relationship. This means the larger the gauge, the smaller the opening.

Length of a Needle

Length is another attribute of a hypodermic needle. Needle length depends on the route of administration. Remember, a needle may be inserted below the skin, into a vein, or deep into thick muscle tissue.

Filters

Filters are often used in combination with needles or other CSP equipment to help prevent or remove contamination. The size of the filter varies according to use.

Filter Needles

Filter needles are molded into the hub of the needle and are designed for one-time use only. They remove glass shards that may contaminate a solution when using a glass ampule.

Filter Straws

A filter straw is a thin, sterile straw with a filter in the hub. Filter straws are used to withdraw a single dose of fluid from a sterile glass ampule.

Vented Needles

Vented needles are used primarily for reconstituting a powdered medication. This type of needle usually has side openings and a thin wall, which act as filters to help minimize spraying and foaming during the reconstitution process.

Dosage Containers

Many sterile products must be administered in small amounts, or doses. For these, the CSP is prepared and stored in a single-dose vial, multiple-dose vial, or an ampule.

Ampules

Ampules are sealed containers made entirely of glass and contain a single dose of medication. Once you open an ampule, it becomes an open system. Remove the single dose and discard the container. Ampules are intended for one-time use only.

When you open an ampule, tiny shards of glass may mix in with the contents. You can extract these unwanted particles by using a filter needle. Remember that you must discard the filter needle after using it.

Single-Dose Vials

Single-dose vials contain one dose of medication and are discarded after one use. For this reason, manufacturers do not add unnecessary preservatives.

The top of a single-dose vial has a rubber stopper. The needle pierces the stopper in order to draw fluid. You must be sure to insert the needle correctly into the stopper, or rubber pieces may break off into the solution, causing contamination.

Multiple-Dose Vials

Multiple-dose vials allow you to access the contents of the vial more than once. This means that the rubber stopper of a multiple-dose vial is punctured more than one time, thereby exposing the contents of the vial to air. Because of this, multiple-dose vials contain preservatives to keep the contents stable.

All vials should be dated and stored according to the manufacturer's requirements. Check stored vials frequently and discard those that are no longer considered stable. Remember that stability is the ability of a CSP to remain effective until used, or until the expiration date has been reached.

Route of Administration

The specific way that a drug comes into contact with body tissue is its route of administration. Usually the physician, physician's assistant, or nurse is responsible for administering a drug. However, it's still important for pharmacy technicians to understand the process of administration. Occasionally, a patient may ask a question about a drug he or she has received. But more importantly, the specific ways in which you prepare certain drugs often depend on the route of administration.

Parenterals

The majority of sterile products that a pharmacy technician will compound are called parenterals. **Parenterals** are simply CSPs that are injected. A parenteral may be injected under the patient's skin or into a joint, the spinal column, a muscle, a vein, an artery, or even the heart. Parenterals are absorbed quickly in areas where the body's defense mechanisms do not have a chance to work. Once administered, a parenteral product cannot be removed. Problems with dose or adverse side effects may be difficult or impossible to reverse.

RECALL TIP

To help remember where an intravenous injection goes, remember the letters IV. The letters IV can stand for **i**ntra-**v**enous, and they can also stand for "**i**nto **v**ein."

Intravenous (IV) Injections

An **intravenous (IV) injection** is one that goes directly into a vein. The type of CSP that is injected is called an intravenous (IV) admixture—a measured substance added to a 50 mL or larger bag or bottle of IV fluid. An intravenous injection is the most common parenteral route of administration.

IV injection is also the fastest parenteral route of administration. Since drug absorption is not a factor, optimum blood levels may be achieved with accuracy and immediacy not possible by other routes. In emergencies, IV administration of a drug may be lifesaving because the drug is placed directly into the circulation.

The parts of an IV system that determine the flow rate of the fluid or medication are called the IV administration set. There are two different types of sets:

- vented set—used for containers that have no venting system (i.e. no IV bags or bottles)
- unvented set—used for containers that have their own venting system

IV administration sets come with various features, including ports for infusing secondary medications and filters for blocking microbes.

The tubing of an IV administration set frequently varies. Some types of tubing are designed to enhance the proper functioning of devices that help regulate the infusion rate. Other tubing is used specifically for continuous or intermittent infusion, or for infusing parenteral nutrition and blood.

There are also two main types of IV bagging:

- large-volume IV bags
- intravenous piggybacks (IVPBs)

Large-Volume Intravenous Bags

A **large-volume IV bag** is sometimes called a large-volume IV drip. These are administered continuously and are often used for fluid replacement or for maintenance of fluids. The IV bag label should include the prescription number, name of the patient, medical record number, name and amount of drug, and expiration date. The bag should hang at least 36 inches above the patient's bed.

Intravenous Piggybacks

The other type of IV bagging, **intravenous piggybacks (IVPB)**, are administered on a set schedule (e.g., twice a day, three times a day). IVPB bags are generally smaller than large-volume IV bags. This makes sense since they are added on, or "piggybacked," to a large-volume IV bag. When a piggyback container is added to an IV, the piggyback container needs to be positioned higher than the primary IV container.

Intravenous Infusion Pumps

When the flow of medication needs to be done automatically, an infusion pump is used. An **infusion pump** is an automatic device used with an IV system for delivering medication at regular intervals in specific quantities.

The pump infuses, or delivers, medication into the IV line according to a preset program. This is much easier than having to administer medication manually at certain intervals round the clock.

Intravenous Administration Sets for Manual Infusion

IV fluids that are administered manually use infusions sets. Infusion sets consist of plastic tubing attached to one end of an IV bag and at the other end a needle or catheter inserted into a blood vessel. There are two basic types of infusion sets:

- microdrip
- macrodrip

To deliver 1 mL of fluid to the patient, 60 drops must fall (60 gtt = 1 mL). Microdrip infusion sets always deliver 60 drops of fluid per milliliter (gtt/mL). With macrodrip sets, amounts per milliliter differ according to the manufacturer. For example, macrodrip sets from Baxter deliver 10 gtt/mL; Abbot sets deliver 15 gtts/mL. The package label or insert will always indicate the drops per milliliter. This information is essential in determining the flow rate of an IV infusion.

One type of macrodrip infusion set is an intravenous push (IVP), which is a small volume of medicine (less than 250 mL) that is injected into a vein and administered over a short period of time.

Catheter Lines

When parenteral administration has to be repeated over time, it often makes sense to use a **catheter**. A catheter is a delivery or drainage tube that is inserted into a vein, artery, or body cavity. Fluids can be drained or injected using a catheter line.

Catheters make repeated parenteral administration much easier since they eliminate the need for multiple punctures. Using a single catheter puncture also makes it easier to reduce the risk of contamination.

Sterile technique is very important when using any type of catheter line. A catheter line could easily serve as a place of entry for contaminating substances. The catheter line itself may also become infected. Therefore, the sterile packaging of catheter lines is critically important.

Total Parenteral Nutrition

Total parenteral nutrition (TPN) or **total nutrition admixture (TNA)** is IV therapy that provides nutrition to patients who cannot take nourishment by mouth. It is composed of the following basic nutrition and fluid components:

- Dextrose: a major source of calories; each gram of dextrose provides 3.4 kcal. It is available in a concentrated form (50% or more) that is diluted in the final TPN solution to approximately 25%.

RECALL TIP

Use the phrase "thorough patient nourishment" to remember what TPN means. This will help you remember that TPN also stands for total parenteral nutrition.

- Amino acids: a source of protein that is required for tissue growth and repair; each gram of protein provides 4 kcal
- Fat: essential fatty acids
- Basic electrolytes: required for metabolic needs and deficiencies, such as potassium chloride

Fat Emulsions

Fat emulsions are used to prevent essential fatty acid depletion (EFAD). They can also be used as a source of calories. The dextrose, amino acids, electrolytes, and fat emulsions are often incorporated into one container. These are referred to as All-in-One or 3-in-1 solutions, or TNAs (total nutrition admixtures). These preparations are infused via a central vein. IV fat emulsions are available as 10, 20, or 30% emulsions. The 30% product is indicated only for administration as part of a 3-in-1 or TNA.

Chapter Summary

- Compound sterile products, or CSPs, are mixtures of one or more substances that are made free of contamination before use.
- CSPs must be prepared in a sterile environment. To minimize contamination, the air is carefully filtered, and access is limited. In addition, technicians must wear protective clothing, gloves and headgear, and use specialized equipment such as laminar airflow workbenches.
- The pieces of equipment used to administer a drug are known as the drug's delivery system. Common delivery system equipment includes syringes, filters, and dosage containers.
- There are many different routes of administration for giving drugs to patients. One frequent route of administration is via injection. Drugs can be injected into the skin, muscle, spinal column, arteries, or veins of a patient.
- Intravenous (IV) injections can be used to deliver many types of CSPs straight into the patient's circulatory system. One common use of IV therapy is total parenteral nutrition (TPN), which provides nutrition to patients who cannot take nourishment by mouth.

PRACTICE TEST QUESTIONS

Sterile Products and Pharmacy Equipment

1. All manipulations inside an LAH should be performed at least ____ inches inside the hood to prevent ____.
   a. 12 inches; smoke
   b. 6 inches; contamination
   c. 10 inches; contamination
   d. 2 inches; breakage from falling on the floor

2. An ampule is composed entirely of glass. Once broken, it:
   a. becomes an open system
   b. remains a closed system
   c. turns into a multiple dose solution
   d. none are correct

3. IV tubing used as a primary set includes which of the following?
   a. macro drop tubing (delivering 10 gtt/min)
   b. micro drip tubing (delivering 60 gtt/min)
   c. all purpose tubing (delivering 100 gtt/min)
   d. both a & b

4. To assure the sterility of a new needle:
   a. wipe the needle with 70% isopropyl to disinfect it
   b. apply additional silicone so the needle self sterilizes upon insertion into a vial
   c. only open the package in a clean room
   d. make sure the package was intact and not damaged

5. IV fluid should hang how many inches higher than the patient's bed?

   a. 12 inches
   b. 24 inches
   c. 36 inches
   d. 49 inches

6. The piggyback is placed _____ the primary IV.

   a. Lower than
   b. higher than
   c. at the same height as
   d. away from

7. Ampules differ from vials in that they:

   a. are closed systems
   b. require the use of a filter needle
   c. can be opened without risk of breakage
   d. do not differ from vials

8. The labeling of an IV admixture should contain all of the following information *except*:

   a. patient name
   b. name and amount of drug(s) added
   c. prescribing physician's name
   d. expiration date

9. Dextrose is the base component of TPN solutions that are most commonly given as a source of carbohydrates. Which of the following statements are true?

   a. Dextrose is available in a concentrated form (50% or more) that is diluted in the final TPN solution to approximately 25%
   b. Dextrose is available as a 5% solution that is commonly used as is in TPN solutions
   c. Dextrose is available as a 70% solution that is commonly given as a separate infusion for calories and energy
   d. all of the above

10. The CADD is an example of what type of pump system?

    a. mechanical system
    b. ambulatory electronic infusion pump system
    c. electronic controlled pressure and chemical release system
    d. none of the above

11. The most common complication of tunneled venous access devices are:

    a. catheter occlusion
    b. infections
    c. dislodgement
    d. venous thrombosis

12. The space between the HEPA filter and the sterile product being prepared is referred to as the:

    a. hot spot
    b. backwash zone
    c. zone of turbulence
    d. critical area

13. Electrolytes are added to TPN solutions to meet metabolic needs and correct deficiencies. Examples of electrolytes include:

    a. potassium chloride
    b. amino acids
    c. vitamin D
    d. lipid emulsions

14. Lipid or fat emulsions are typically administered by all of the following methods *except*:

    a. as a 10% emulsion given through a peripheral line
    b. as a 20% emulsion given through a peripheral line
    c. as part of an IV push
    d. as part of a 3-in-1 solution

15. Preservatives in parenteral products:

    a. kill organisms and eliminate the need for aseptic technique and LAHs
    b. are present in multi-dose vials
    c. are harmless and non-toxic in any amount
    d. all of the above are correct

16. Items inside an LAH should be placed away from other objects and the walls of the hood to prevent:

    a. zones of turbulence
    b. windows of contamination
    c. dead space
    d. laminar air zones

17. Mixing of 3-in-1 solutions should be performed carefully to prevent the emulsion from "oiling out." It is recommended that this be accomplished by:

    a. preparing the solution in a very cold room
    b. preparing the solution from fresh lipids
    c. using a mixing order of fats, amino acids, and dextrose
    d. using a mixing order of dextrose, fats, and then amino acids

18. After a cytotoxic agent is prepared in the pharmacy, transportation:

    a. should be done immediately
    b. should be done in a way as to minimize breakage
    c. includes making the transporter aware of what they are carrying and what the procedure would be in the event of a spill
    d. both b & c

19. Protective apparel for those preparing cytotoxic or hazardous injections in a BSC includes:
    a. a low permeability, solid front gown with tight fitting elastic cuffs
    b. latex gloves
    c. a self-contained respirator
    d. both a & b

20. Needle sizes are described by two numbers. The ___ corresponds to the diameter of its bore. The ____ measures the shaft.
    a. length; gauge
    b. gauge; length
    c. gauge; tip
    d. depth; length

21. Human touch contamination is the most common source of IV related contamination.
    a. true
    b. false

22. There are two types of area used for compounding in the home care setting. The area that is controlled for microorganisms within designated specifications is called:
    a. sterile compounding area
    b. clean compounding area
    c. bacteria free area
    d. clean room

23. Sterile products should be prepared in a "class 100" environment. In most pharmacies this is accomplished with the use of a:
    a. room air filter
    b. fan cycling air 100 times per hour
    c. laminar Air Flow Hood (LAH)
    d. fume hood

24. In the typical IV setup, an LVP is attached to a primary set, which is then attached to the catheter and inserted into the patient. Drugs administered intermittently are usually given:
    a. through a Y-site injection port or flashball on the primary set
    b. by adding them to the LVP solution
    c. through another IV line (not through the one used for the LVP)
    d. through the same site as the primary IV

25. Large volume parenteral solution containers with potent drugs that need to be infused with a high degree of accuracy and precision are usually administered with the aid of a:
    a. roller clamp
    b. electronic infusion device
    c. hand clamp
    d. counting device controlled by the nurse

Preparation of Non-Sterile Products

Test Topics

After completing this chapter, you should be able to demonstrate knowledge of the following:

1. Procedures to prepare oral dosage forms in unit-dose or non–unit-dose packaging
2. Procedures to compound non-sterile products
3. Procedures to prepare ready-to-dispense multidose packages

Test Terms

- **Class A prescription balance scale** scale required by law for use in the pharmacy to weigh out dosages of solid medications
- **Food and Drug Administration (FDA)** agency of the United States government that controls the drugs that are acceptable for use in the United States
- **Drug Enforcement Administration (DEA)** agency of the United States government that controls who may prescribe, distribute, and fill prescriptions for controlled or scheduled drugs in the United States
- **levigation** process to reduce particle size and grittiness of added powders for small scale preparation of ointments
- **multidose packaging system** drug packaging system in which medication is distributed in single-dose packing but where the dose is more than one unit
- **non-unit-dose distribution system** drug packaging system in which medication is distributed in bulk bottles
- **solubility** the property of a substance that can be dissolved in a liquid to form a homogenous solution
- **solutions** drugs that are dissolved in liquid; the most common solvent is water
- **suspensions** drugs that have been finely divided and placed in a liquid or fluid vehicle; oral suspensions are usually water-based, but suspensions intended for other purposes can have different vehicles
- **unit dose distribution system** drug packaging system in which medication is distributed in single-dose packaging
- **United States Pharmacopeia (USP)** non-governmental, official public standard-setting authority for prescription and over-the-counter medicines and other healthcare products manufactured or sold in the United States.

As a pharmacy technician, you will be required to prepare drugs for your patients. Many of these drugs are non-sterile. Like the methods required in preparing sterile products, the procedures to prepare non-sterile medicines are relatively easy to follow. Knowing how to properly prepare oral dosage medication, non-sterile compounds, and ready-to-dispense packages will help make you a qualified and capable pharmacy technician.

Most hospitals dispense medication to patients using the **unit dose distribution system**. This packaging system allows the medication to be dispensed in a single-dose package ready to be administered to the patient. The label on the package includes the name of the drug (both brand and generic if applicable), the dosage strength, and the expiration date. This type of system is considered safer for patients because there is less opportunity for medication distribution errors.

In most community pharmacies, **non-unit-dose systems**, in which medication is distributed in bulk bottles, are the norm.

Multidose packaging distribution systems distributes the medication in packages that contain the number of tablets or capsules per dose. The patient may be required to take two tablets for one dose; this type of system dispenses the proper number of tablets per dose.

Government Regulators

Before getting into the details of administering and preparing medications, it is important to know that there are two federal agencies responsible for regulating the drugs you will be working with. **The Food and Drug Administration (FDA)** controls the drugs that are acceptable for use in the United States. The **Drug Enforcement Administration (DEA)** controls who may prescribe, distribute, and fill prescriptions for controlled or scheduled drugs.

The FDA is primarily responsible for regulating the safety of prescription and non-prescription drugs in the United States. The Federal Food, Drug, and Cosmetic Act states that before a new drug can enter the market, it must be approved by the FDA. The pharmaceutical company developing the drug must provide empirical evidence that its product is safe and effective. The administration is also responsible for regulating the safety and efficacy of generic and over-the-counter drugs as well. In keeping with their mission to ensure that all drugs in the United States meet the minimum safety requirements, the FDA is responsible for establishing and enforcing the guidelines that regulate manufacturers that package and distribute medications. These guidelines, known as the Current Good Manufacturing Practice (cGMP), establish the requirements for all aspects of pharmaceutical manufacturing. The FDA enforces these regulations by conducting inspections of the facilities and production logs of the pharmaceutical companies.

Routes of Administration

There are many different ways to administer medication to a patient. Usually, these routes are chosen by the physician after he or she considers several factors. These factors include:

- cost
- safety
- effectiveness

Oral Dosage Forms

The most common route of administering medication is oral. Oral dosage medication is taken through the mouth. Examples include tablets, capsules, and liquids. The majority of medications found in a typical person's nightstand drawer or medicine cabinet are probably in oral dosage form. As a pharmacy technician, it will be part of your job to prepare and dispense these types of medication. Let's take a closer look at the three most common forms of oral medicine: tablets, capsules, and suspensions.

Capsules and Tablets

Tablets are solid dosage forms that have been compressed or molded. Tablets can come with or without diluents (or fillers), disintegrants (used to separate certain ingredients), coatings (used to protect the tablet from external factors like moisture and stomach acid), and colorants (often used by commercial companies to "brand" their tablets).

Capsules are solid dosage forms in which the drug ingredients and fillers are enclosed in a gelatinous shell. Capsules can be of any size and are often distinctive in shape and color. Because a capsule's shell dissolves rapidly, the drugs inside a capsule are released much faster than tablets. The method a technician uses to fill a capsule is the known as the punch method. The punch method consists of placing the powder on a compounding slab, also known as an ointment slab, and smoothing it with a spatula to a height approximately half the length of the capsule body. The bottom of the capsule is held vertically and the open end is repeatedly punched into the powder until the capsule has reached full capacity, and then the top is placed on the capsule.

Capsules come in many different sizes: 000, 00, 0, 1, 2, 3, 4, and 5. The higher the number of the capsule, the less volume it can hold. For example, a size 5 capsule can hold less of a drug than a size 1 capsule.

Liquid Medicines

Suspensions are drugs that have been finely divided and placed in some sort of liquid or fluid vehicle. Oral suspensions are usually water-based, but suspensions intended for other purposes can have different vehicles. (For example, drugs that are injected intramuscularly are maintained in oil rather than water.) In order to form a suspension, the drug particles should be insoluble. This is why suspensions are shaken before they are used. The particles that have settled will be more evenly distributed after shaking, which ensures that the proper dosage will be taken. In fact, a technician who prepares a suspension must place an auxiliary label on the container that reads "Shake Well." Suspensions are absorbed by the body faster than capsules since they are presented in finer particle size and are ready for dissolution immediately upon ingestion.

Oral Solutions

Solutions are the most commonly compounded drug dosage form. Drugs that are administered in an aqueous, or water-based, solution are most rapidly absorbed because they don't require dissolution or disintegration. While the most common solvent is water, any ingredient that is dissolved in a solution can change its fluidity if different liquids are used. For example, an elixir uses a sweetened hydroalcohol as its main solvent, while a syrup generally uses a sucrose solution. These flavorants and colorants are added to oral solutions in order to make the medicine easier to take. Sometimes, these additives are necessary to maintain the chemical and physical properties of the medication. If no other preservatives are present, solutions require a minimum of about 15% of alcohol to ensure that the medicine is properly preserved.

Solubility

Solubility is the property of a substance that can be dissolved in a liquid to form a homogenous solution. It is measured as amount of solute concentrated in a liquid, or solvent, when equilibrium is reached. When a solvent at a given temperature has dissolved all of the solute it can, the result is called a saturated solution.

Powders

The term *powder* can mean several different things in the world of pharmacology. On the one hand, when a drug is a dry substance made up of finely divided particles, the word *powder* refers to the drug's physical form. *Powder* can also be used to describe a type of pharmaceutical preparation for internal or external use. In either case, powders are mixtures of dry, finely divided drugs or chemicals that can be used either internally or externally. Powders are very versatile drugs. They can be fabricated into solid dosage forms like tablets and caplets, dissolved or suspended in solvents to make liquid dosage forms, or formulated into medicated ointments and creams.

Analyzing Particle Size

Pharmaceutical powders have a varied range of size and texture, from a relatively coarse 10mm diameter, to an extremely fine size of one micron or less. The **United States Pharmacopeia (USP)** characterizes a powder's particle size into the following categories:

- very coarse
- coarse
- moderately coarse
- fine
- very fine

These descriptions are all based on the proportion of powder that can pass through the openings of a mechanical sieve shaker. Sieves have standard openings that determine how fine a powder or granule is (see the following table).

Opening of Standard Sieves	
Sieve Number	**Sieve Opening**
2.0	9.50mm
3.5	5.60mm
4.0	4.75mm
8.0	2.36mm
10.0	2.00mm
20.0	850.00μm
30.0	600.00μm
40.0	425.00μm
50.0	300.00μm

(continued)

Opening of Standard Sieves *(continued)*	
Sieve Number	**Sieve Opening**
60.0	250.00μm
70.0	212.00μm
80.0	180.00μm
100.0	150.00μm
120.0	125.00μm
200.0	75.00μm
230.0	63.00μm
270.0	53.00μm
325.0	45.00μm
400.0	38.00μm

The purpose of a particle size analysis in pharmacology is to obtain data on the size, distribution, and shape of drugs being used in pharmaceutical formulations. Determining particle size can influence several characteristics of drugs, including:

- the dissolution rate at which particles dissolve
- the suspendability of undissolved particles dispersed in a liquid
- the uniform distribution of drugs in a powder mixture
- the penetrability of particles intended for inhalation
- the level of grittiness in dermal ointments and creams

Levigation

Levigation is commonly used in small scale preparation of ointments to reduce the particle size and grittiness of added powders. A mortar and pestle is used for this process. When using a mortar and pestle to combine substances, the most potent ingredient, or the ingredient that is used in the smallest amount, is placed in the mortar first. A paste is formed by combining the insoluble powder and a small amount of liquid, which is the levigating agent. This paste is then triturated, reducing particle size. The levigated paste is added to the ointment base and the mixture is made uniform and smooth by rubbing them together. There are different types of mortar and pestle used to mix different substances. In order to mix a suspension or a porous liquid, a glass mortar and pestle must be used.

Measurement Devices

Measuring medications is a delicate process, as a minor mistake in dosage could cause severe, or even lethal, consequences in a patient. Balance scales are used in the pharmacy to weigh out dosages of solid medications. It is actually required by law that a pharmacy has a **Class A prescription balance scale** on hand for dosage measurement.

The minimum weight that a Class A scale can measure is 120 mg, in order to avoid weighing errors of 5% or greater. When operating a prescription balance scale, a technician must use a pair of tweezers to avoid altering the weight of the metal. The slightest touch of the scale could cause an imbalance that might endanger a patient's life. Weights are used on balance scale to balance the amount of drug with the amount of weight on the scale. The weights must always be placed on the right side of the scale. In order to determine the exact weight of a drug, the scale must be at a point of zero balance, or equilibrium.

The primary instrument for measuring medications in liquid form is a graduate. A graduate is defined as a calibrated measuring container used to mix liquids. There are two types of graduates used in pharmacy; conical and cylindrical. Cylindrical graduates are typically calibrated in metric units, and conical graduates may be calibrated to both metric and apothecary units. When measuring a liquid, it is important to choose a graduate appropriate to the amount of medication being measured. Liquid should be poured into the graduate slowly, and always at eye level. For accuracy, the liquid should be measured at the bottom of the meniscus.

Chapter Summary

- The FDA is primarily responsible for regulating the safety of prescription and non-prescription drugs in the United States.
- The most common route of administering medication is oral. Examples include tablets, capsules, and liquids.
- Measuring medications is a delicate process, as a minor mistake in dosage could cause severe negative consequences in a patient, even death.
- Solubility occurs when a multi-component liquid is able to dissolve a substance, or solute, at a specific temperature and pressure.
- The purpose of a particle size analysis in pharmacology is to obtain data on the size, distribution, and shape of drugs being used in pharmaceutical formulations.
- Levigation is commonly used in small scale preparation of ointments to reduce the particle size and grittiness of added powders.

PRACTICE TEST QUESTIONS

Preparation of Non-Sterile Products

1. The most commonly compounded formulations are:
   a. ointment
   b. tablets
   c. solutions
   d. lotions

2. The most common solvent for oral solutions is:
   a. alcohol
   b. glycerin
   c. syrups
   d. water

3. The minimum amount of alcohol required to preserve solutions if no other preservatives are present is:
   a. 15%
   b. 20%
   c. 25%
   d. 30%

4. Which of the steps listed below is part of the process of preparing an oral suspension from a tablet?
   a. powdering of tablets with a mortar and pestle
   b. wet the powder to make a paste
   c. dilute the wet powder to the desired concentration
   d. all of the above

5. Which of the following results in the most wasted product:
   a. extemporaneous
   b. repackaging
   c. batching
   d. none of the above

6. The expiration date given to oral solids that are repackaged is:

    a. One year from the date of repackaging
    b. Six months from the date of repackaging or 25% of the remaining time between the date of repackaging and the expiration date of the oral solid
    c. Six months from the date of repackaging
    d. 25% of the remaining time between the date of repackaging and the expiration date of the oral solid

7. The organization responsible for providing the guidelines for manufacturers that package medications is the:

    a. Drug Enforcement Agency
    b. Bureau of Manufacturers
    c. The United States Pharmacopeia
    d. Food and Drug Administration

8. Scales differ in their range of weight. When weighing 150 mg of medication, the technician should use:

    a. a class A balance
    b. a class B balance
    c. a class C balance
    d. either a class A or B balance

9. A graduate is defined as:

    a. a concave container used to mix liquids
    b. a calibrated measuring container used to mix liquids
    c. a container used to mix larger products that require high-speed blending
    d. instrument used to stir products such as suspensions

10. The weights of a balance are very sensitive. The technician must use tweezers to prevent:

    a. improper measurement of medication
    b. offsetting the measurement of medication
    c. altering the exact weight of the metal
    d. prevent oils from the hands getting onto the metal

11. Of the information listed below, which one is not required to apply on the label of a unit dose item?

    a. name of the drug
    b. dosage strength
    c. expiration date
    d. patient's name

12. The definition of levigation is:

    a. triturating a powder drug with a solvent in which it is insoluble to reduce its particle size.
    b. the fine grinding of a powder
    c. a technique for mixing two powders of unequal size
    d. fully and evenly combining a mixture

13. When a solution at room temperature has absorbed all of the solute it can, it is called a:

    a. supersaturated solution
    b. complete solution
    c. saturated solution
    d. soluble solution

14. Of the following capsules, which one would hold the least volume?

    a. size 0
    b. size 1
    c. size 4
    d. size 5

15. The method a technician uses to fill a capsule is called the:

    a. slide method
    b. punch method
    c. fill method
    d. cake method

16. When combining drugs in a mortar and pestle, the most potent ingredient or the ingredient that occurs in the smallest amount is placed in the mortar:

    a. first
    b. last
    c. part of the medication at the beginning and part at the end
    d. in small amounts throughout the process

17. An ingredient dissolved in a solution is known as a:

    a. solute
    b. solvent
    c. suspension
    d. emulsion

18. In order to _____, a suppository-forming liquid is immediately poured into a mold.

    a. prevent contamination
    b. mix the ingredients
    c. prevent exposure to the air
    d. solidify the suppository

19. When placing weights on a balance, they should always be placed:

    a. on the right hand side
    b. on the left hand side
    c. using a spatula
    d. with gloves

20. When measuring small amount of liquid, it is best to use a:

    a. cylindrical graduate
    b. conical graduate
    c. pipette
    d. medicine dropper

21. The zero point of a balance scale is called:
    a. equal point
    b. equilibrium
    c. levigation
    d. counter balance

22. A compounding slab is also called a:
    a. porcelain slab
    b. clean slab
    c. sterile slab
    d. ointment slab

23. When preparing a suspension, an auxiliary label should be applied to the container that states:
    a. Take only with food
    b. Take on an empty stomach
    c. Shake Well
    d. Take with a large amount of water

24. While pouring a liquid slowly into a graduate, the measurement should be:
    a. observed on eye level
    b. observed by looking down into the graduate
    c. reading the level of the liquid from the top of the meniscus
    d. all of the above are acceptable

25. The type of mortar and pestle used to mix suspensions or porous liquids is:
    a. porcelain
    b. glass
    c. plastic
    d. china

10

Dispensing Medications

There are several government agencies that regulate drug activity.

- The **Food and Drug Administration (FDA)** regulates drugs that are acceptable for use in the United States.

- The **Drug Enforcement Administration (DEA)** regulates controlled substances, their schedule, and who can use them.

- The U.S. Boards of Pharmacy regulate pharmacy practice including distribution, sale, and storage of pharmaceuticals.

Each state has a separate board of pharmacy that may enforce activities differently. Therefore, in addition to closely following the guidelines in your work setting, you should contact your state board for specific regulations.

Dispensing medications involves a variety of considerations including everything from specific site practices to customer service procedures. You must understand several aspects of quality control such as drug errors, forged prescriptions, record-keeping, and accurate labeling. It's also important for pharmacy technicians to understand legal issues such as the five categories of controlled substances, restrictions on drug counseling, and refill requirements.

Dispensing Drugs

Dispensing a drug involves preparing and distributing a medication to a patient. Only pharmacists, pharmacy technicians, physicians, properly credentialed nurse practitioners, and physicians' assistants may dispense drugs.

Prescription Information

You need vital information before you can fill a patient's prescription, including:

- physician's name, address, and phone number
- date of prescription
- patient's name, address, and phone number
- drug, dose, and form
- number of doses
- number of refills
- insurance number or medical record number
- signa or sig (instructions to the patient on how to take the medication)
- DEA number
- physician's signature
- DAW ("dispense as written," meaning a generic drug cannot be substituted for the brand name drug indicated on the prescription form)

In addition to information that you'll find on the prescription order, it's a good idea to have a patient's demographic information, allergies to medications, and any third-party insurance information.

To process a prescription, the insurance company will need:

- the name of the insured (cardholder)
- group number
- identification number
- dependent information (i.e., who is covered—spouse, children, etc.)
- expiration date of coverage
- co-pay amount paid by patient
- carrier (name of the provider of pharmacy service)

Prescription Labels

Federal law requires that certain information appear on prescription labels, including:

- name of the patient
- name and address of the pharmacy

- prescription serial number
- date of the prescription or refill
- name of the prescriber
- directions for use with precautions

Prescription Errors

Prescription errors are common. You should be mindful of mistakes in the following areas:

- abnormal doses
- early refills
- incorrect drugs
- wrong strength of drugs
- incorrect patient IDs
- forged orders

Filling Prescription Orders

As a pharmacy technician, you can help avoid incorrect prescriptions. You should carry out the following procedures each time you fill a prescription to reduce errors:

- Check the drug three times: when taking out the drug container, after placing the medication in the dispenser, and before returning the drug container to storage.
- Verify the route and dose that the physician ordered with the route and dose you prepared.
- Check when and how the patient should take the medication (e.g., now, two times a day, with meals, etc).
- Document the procedure in the patient's medical record: note the date, time, drug, dose, route, site, results/tolerance, and patient education.
- Verify the name on the physician's order.
- Ensure that the pharmacist does a final check of the prescription.

Detecting Forged Medication Orders

It's vital for you to assure that every prescription you fill is not altered or forged. You do this by:

- checking prescription indications against those found on the drug's package insert
- checking the patient's ID
- remaining alert to the number of prescriptions a prescriber writes in comparison to other practitioners in the area
- double checking handwritten orders or orders written in the names of other people
- checking the Drug Enforcement Administration (DEA) number

If you believe a patient has forged a prescription, notify the pharmacist, so he or she can call the doctor to verify the legitimacy of the prescription. If the prescription is verified as a forgery, the pharmacist should call the local police station.

DEA Registration Numbers

The DEA registration number should appear on every prescription as a way to track the delivery of controlled substances. The first letter of a DEA number reflects the prescriber's practice. The second letter is the first letter of the prescriber's last name. The seven numbers are determined by adding the first, third, and fifth number (odd group). Add the second, fourth, and sixth number (even group) and multiply by two. Add the two sums together. The final number should match the last digit of the DEA number. Let's use DEA number BT1197967 as an example.

1. Add the odd group: $1 + 9 + 9 = 19$
2. Add the even group and multiply the answer by 2: $1 + 7 + 6 = 14 \times 2 = 28$
3. Add the two sums together: $28 + 19 = 47$
4. The last digit is the same as the last digit of the DEA number.

Controlled Substances

The DEA has created the **Schedule of Controlled Substances,** which organizes certain drugs according to their tendencies to cause dependence and abuse. There are five categories:

- *Schedule I.* These substances have no accepted medicinal uses in the United States.
- *Schedule II.* These drugs carry severe restrictions. Dispensing these drugs requires a written prescription, which cannot be refilled or called into a pharmacy by the medical office. The physician may only call in an order to a pharmacy in extreme emergencies for up to a 72-hour dose, and patients must present the original written and signed prescription to the pharmacist within seven days of the call.
- *Schedule III.* A physician may call the prescription into the pharmacy. The order can be refilled up to five times in six months.
- *Schedule IV.* A medical office employee may call the prescription into the pharmacy. The order can be refilled up to five times in six months.
- *Schedule V.* These are drugs with accepted medical use with a low potential for abuse.

Schedule II prescriptions cannot be transferred between pharmacies. However, a patient can transfer among pharmacies controlled substances III-V the amount of times that they are refillable as long as the pharmacies share an electronic real-time database. Also, state law may require that all drugs contain a "federal transfer label" stating that "federal law prohibits the transfer of the drug to any person other than the patient for whom it was prescribed."

Individual state laws may vary on how you handle controlled drugs. For example, not all states consider Schedule V drugs as OTC medications, other restrictions may apply on refills, and so on.

See the following table for some examples of each type of controlled substance.

> **RECALL TIP**
>
> There's a lot to remember when it comes to controlled substances. But it's easy if you think of them in terms of patients climbing up a ladder. Each rung up is a step toward easier restrictions on the Schedule of Controlled Substances. For example, if a patient takes a Schedule II drug, there is high risk involved and more adverse reactions, therefore, he shouldn't climb as high. If another patient takes a Schedule V drug, there is less risk involved and fewer adverse reactions, so she can climb higher.

Investigational Drugs

> **RECALL TIP**
>
> Remember that *investigational* drugs are still being *investigated* by the FDA to determine their safety and effectiveness. For this reason, these drugs carry some additional restrictions.

Investigational drugs are substances the FDA has not yet approved for human use. These drugs are used in clinical trials. A pharmacy may only dispense investigational drugs under special circumstances in which the prescribing physician provides written permission from the study sponsor. Investigational drugs must be kept separate from other drugs in the pharmacy and a record of use must be kept. Also, these drugs cannot be exchanged among patients on the same medication. Each patient must have her own supply. The unused portion of investigational drugs should be returned to the manufacturer if they expire or if the medication is discontinued by the provider.

Over-the-Counter Drugs

Over-the-counter (OTC) drugs are available in pharmacies without any restrictions. The label of an OTC drug must contain the manufacturer's name, expiration date, and the established name of all active ingredients.

Schedule of Controlled Substances

Schedule	Potential for Abuse	Examples
Schedule I (C-I)	High potential for abuse No acceptable medical use in the United States	heroin marijuana LSD (lysergic acid diethylamide) peyote
Schedule II (C-II)	Potential for high abuse with severe physical or psychological dependence	narcotics such as meperidine, methadone, morphine, and oxycodone amphetamines barbiturates
Schedule III (C-III)	Less potential for abuse than Schedule II drugs Potential for moderate physical or psychological dependence	nonbarbiturate sedatives nonamphetamine stimulants limited amounts of certain narcotics aspirin, butalbital, caffeine, and codeine (Fiorinal with Codeine) paregoric (Camphorated Tincture of Opium)
Schedule IV (C-IV)	Less potential for abuse than Schedule III drugs Limited potential for dependence	some sedatives and anxiety medications nonnarcotic analgesics (painkillers) valium (Diastat, Diazepam Intensol, Valium) midazolam (Versed, Versed Syrup) zolpidem (Ambien, Ambien CR)
Schedule V (C-V)	Limited potential for abuse	small amounts of narcotics (codeine) used to control coughing (antitussives) or diarrhea (antidiarrheals)

Effects of Disabilities on Drug and Non-Drug Therapy

Some patients have challenges to overcome before they can comply with their drug and non-drug therapy. Assessing patients' cognitive abilities is especially important when the pharmacist gives them information about adverse reactions and dosage regimen. Their safety depends on their understanding of the drug. This can be done by evaluating a patient's:

- reading ability
- learning impairments
- communication skills
- education level

Patients with hearing impairments may require you to use simple sentences and vocabulary in order to read your lips. The patient may also use a different type of communication, such as an interpreter, teletypewriters (TTY), or telecommunications devices (TDD), so it's a good idea to familiarize yourself with these devices.

For some visually impaired patients, you may need to simply use bright-colored stickers to differentiate medication. For others, it may be necessary to vary the size of medication bottles so patients can identify the medication.

RECALL TIP

When assessing a patient's cognitive abilities, remember the acronym *CLEAR*:

- C communication skills
- L learning impairments
- E education level
- AR ability to read

Chapter Summary

- Dispensing a drug involves preparing and distributing a medication to a patient.
- A prescription cannot be filled without patient, physician, and dosage information.
- Drugs should be checked three times when filled: when the drug is taken out of a container, when it is placed in a dispenser, and when it is returned to the storage container.
- The route, dose, time, method, and physician's name should be checked each time a prescription is filled.
- There are many ways to detect a forged prescription, including verifying the prescriber's DEA number.
- The DEA is responsible for maintaining the list of drugs on the Schedule of Controlled Substances; there are five categories.
- Investigational drugs are drugs under trial and are not approved for human use.
- Over-the-counter drugs do not require a prescription; the label must include the manufacture's name, expiration date, and all of the ingredients.
- Customer service in the pharmacy includes providing patients with any information they request in regard to their medication.
- Age, cultural background, education, comprehension level, occupation, and developmental difficulties can create challenges to drug and non-drug therapy.
- Potential challenges must be considered when patients are given instructions for a prescription.

PRACTICE TEST QUESTIONS

Dispensing Medications

1. The automatic stop date for antibiotics is:
   a. one week.
   b. two weeks.
   c. three weeks.
   d. determined by the prescribing physician.

2. Which of the following is an illegal activity for a pharmacy technician?
   a. obtaining laboratory results
   b. providing counseling for a patient
   c. screening orders for nonformulary/restricted drugs
   d. taking medication orders from a medical office

3. Which of the following is NOT required for authorization to release patient information?
   a. a hand-written copy
   b. a signature
   c. a list of the patient's medications
   d. a reason for release

4. Which of the following may need to be labeled with a federal "transfer warning"?
   a. schedule III drugs
   b. schedule IV drugs
   c. schedule V drugs
   d. All of the above

Schedule V controlled substances are considered OTC. They are classified as a scheduled drug because they contain a form of:
   a. Demerol.
   b. morphine.
   c. codeine.
   d. oxycodone.

5. Of the information listed below, which is vital before you can fill a patient's prescription?
   a. address
   b. full name
   c. insurance number or medical record number
   d. all of the above

6. What is the maximum number of refills for a Schedule II prescription order?

   a. six months or five refills
   b. as many refills as the physician indicates
   c. twice a year
   d. no refills

7. What should a pharmacist look for when determining the validity of a prescription?

   a. an indication not found in the package insert
   b. significantly more orders from one prescriber compared to others in the prescriber's area
   c. prescription orders written in the names of other people
   d. all of the above

8. What is the maximum number of refills that you can dispense for a Schedule IV prescription order?

   a. none
   b. one refill within one month from the date written
   c. five refills within six months from the date written
   d. unlimited refills within one year

9. How many times can a patient transfer among pharmacies a refillable prescription for a Schedule III or IV controlled substance?

   a. as many times as the prescription is refillable if the pharmacies share an electronic real-time database
   b. three times between non-related, non-networked pharmacies
   c. as often as the patient and prescriber agree
   d. controlled substances are non-transferable

10. A prescription label must contain all of the following information EXCEPT the:

    a. name and address of the pharmacy.
    b. name of the prescriber.
    c. directions for use with precautions.
    d. time it was filled.

11. One way to detect a forged prescription is to check to see if the:

    a. prescription is folded.
    b. prescription was written several days ago.
    c. directions are written with no abbreviations used.
    d. indications on the description match those of the package insert.

12. How long of a supply can you give, under the pharmacist's discretion, for an emergency refill of a Schedule II medication?

    a. 72 hours
    b. 24 hours
    c. one week
    d. none—refills without authorization is illegal

13. You should perform all the following prevention techniques EXCEPT:

    a. knowing the prescriber's DEA number.
    b. calling the prescriber for verification after dispensing the medication.
    c. asking for proper identification.
    d. calling the doctor if you believe the patient has forged a prescription.

14. Which of the following must be on the label of an over-the-counter medication container?

    a. manufacturer's name
    b. expiration date
    c. established name of all active ingredients
    d. all of the above

15. Investigational drugs are drugs that:

    a. have recently received approval from the FDA for human use.
    b. have not received approval from the FDA for human use.
    c. do not require approval from the FDA.
    d. are only available for terminally ill patients.

16. You can assess a customer's ability to learn by evaluating all of the following EXCEPT:

    a. if the patient has a learning impairment.
    b. if the patient is left-handed or right-handed.
    c. if the patient has difficulty reading.
    d. the education level of the patient.

17. Which of the following is an accurate description of how the DEA assigns an identity to a prescriber?

    a. The DEA randomly assigns a number.
    b. The first two letters are the prescriber's initials. The numbers are randomly assigned.
    c. The first letter determines the prescriber's practice. The second letter is the first letter of the prescriber's last name. The seven numbers are determined by adding the first, third, and fifth number. Add the second, fourth, and sixth number and multiply by two. Add the two sums together. The final number should match the last digit of the DEA number.
    d. The first two letters are the prescriber's initials. The seven numbers are determined by the first six numbers. The last digit should match the last digit of the DEA number.

18. Which of the following patients would benefit from medication bottles that come in different shapes and sizes?

    a. an elderly patient
    b. a hearing-impaired patient
    c. a visually-impaired patient
    d. a patient with a different cultural background

PART 2

Maintaining Medication and Inventory Control Systems

CHAPTER 11 / Inventory Management and Handling and Storage of Medications

11

Inventory Management and Handling and Storage of Medications

Test Topics

After completing this chapter, you should be able to demonstrate knowledge of the following:

1. Proper storage conditions, packaging requirements, and handling for hazardous materials and compounded medications; an explanation of lot numbers and expirations, information for prescription or medication order labels, and drug stability

2. NDC number components

3. Requirements regarding auxiliary labels

4. Requirements regarding patient package inserts

5. Physical and chemical incompatibilities

6. Drug product laws and regulations and professional standards related to obtaining medication supplies, durable medical equipment, and products

7. Pharmaceutical industry procedures for obtaining pharmaceuticals; also purchasing policies, procedures, and practices

8. Formulary or approved stock list

9. Par and reorder levels and drug usage; also inventory receiving process

10. Bioavailability standards

11. The use of DEA controlled substance ordering forms

12. Regulatory requirements regarding record-keeping for repackaged products, recalled products, and refunded products

13. Policies, procedures, and practices for inventory systems

14. Risk management opportunities

15. The FDA's classifications of recalls; systems to identify and return expired and unsalable products; rules and regulations for the removal and disposal of products

16. Legal and regulatory requirements and professional standards governing operations of pharmacies; also

Test Terms

- **formulary** a list of approved drug products stocked by a pharmacy
- **inventory** the quantity and type of substances on hand in the pharmacy
- **manufacturer recalls** occur when there is a problem in the manufacture or distribution of a drug product that may present a risk to public health
- **Material Safety Data Sheets (MSDS)** forms containing data regarding the properties of particular substances
- **National Drug Code (NDC)** the unique numerical code assigned by manufacturers to each drug they produce
- **Occupational Safety and Health Administration (OSHA)** government agency within the United States Department of Labor responsible for maintaining safe and healthy work environments
- **par levels** predetermined quantities of medications that should be kept in stock
- **perpetual inventory** a method to manage the stock of controlled substances on a continuous basis wherein each time a controlled substance is received or dispensed, it is recorded in a computerized system
- **reorder point** the quantity at which a product should be reordered to maintain minimum acceptable quantity in the pharmacy

legal and regulatory requirements and professional standards for preparing, labeling, dispensing, distributing, and administering medications

17. Medication distribution and control systems requirements for the use of medications in various practice settings

18. Medication distribution and control systems requirements for controlled substances, investigational drugs, and hazardous materials and wastes

19. The written, oral, and electronic communication channels necessary to ensure appropriate follow-up and problem resolution

20. Quality assurance policies, procedures, and practices for medication and inventory control systems

As a pharmacy technician, you will likely play a key role in managing inventory. As a result, knowledge of inventory procedures and methods, protocols for drug labeling, and requirements specific to controlled substances and over-the-counter medications will be necessary.

Basic Terms

RECALL TIP

When learning the term *par level*, remember that *par* refers to an accepted standard, or the amount considered the norm.

Inventory refers to the quantity and type of substances on hand. When you take inventory at a pharmacy, you conduct a physical count of all medications in possession. Part of managing inventory at a pharmacy is ensuring that par levels of pharmaceutical products are maintained. **Par levels** are predetermined quantities of medications that should be kept in stock. In addition, pharmacies typically define a minimum quantity that they want in stock, as well as a maximum quantity that they don't want to exceed for a given medication. The **reorder point** refers to quantity at which a product should be reordered to maintain this balance.

Formularies

Pharmaceutical data is maintained in a **formulary**, which is a list of approved drug products stocked by a pharmacy. In a closed formulary, only the drugs on the list will be covered by the insurance company. In an open formulary, the insurance plan may cover drugs that are not on the approved list. Because they are convenient and maintain the most current product information in a purchasing and inventory system, computerized formularies are used in most pharmacies. Formularies are typically updated every 12–18 months. Keep in mind that prescriptions come into the pharmacy by phone, by fax, and, most commonly, through walk-ins. As a result, much of controlling inventory depends on consistently and accurately transferring data into computerized systems, including formularies.

Hazardous Materials

RECALL TIP

Remember that the Occupational Safety and Health Administration is commonly referred to by its acronym, OSHA.

By mandate of the **Occupational Safety and Health Administration (OSHA)**, pharmacies must maintain an inventory of all hazardous materials in the workplace. As part of this, for all hazardous materials there must be **Material Safety Data Sheets (MSDS)** on hand and accessible to employees at all times. MSDS are forms containing data regarding the properties of particular substances.

Inventory Procedures and Methods

Effective management of pharmaceutical inventory requires that invoices for purchases be kept to document the receipt of drug orders from manufacturers to the pharmacy. If the purchase order or manufacturer's invoice cannot be located, then the date of receipt, name of receiver, product name, strength, dosage form, and amount should all be recorded and filed in pharmacy records.

Inventory Adjustments

Various situations may require adjustment of a pharmacy's inventory level on a short-term basis or long-term basis. For example, increased need for products such as asthma medication during allergy seasons, or treating a patient who requires an unusually high dose of a given medication, would make short-term inventory adjustments necessary. In contrast, the increased use of a particular product by multiple patients over the course of several months may indicate a need for long-term inventory adjustments, such as an increase in inventory requirements.

Storage of Medications

RECALL TIP

To convert Celsius temperatures to Fahrenheit temperatures, or Fahrenheit to Celsius, use the following formulas:

- Celsius to Fahrenheit:
  $(°C \times 1.8) + 32 = °F$
- Fahrenheit to Celsius:
  $(°F - 32) \times 0.56 = °C$

Temperature is critical for the storage of medications. Most medications need to be stored at room temperature, which is 15° to 30° C, or 59° to 86°F. In addition, there are a variety of storage methods, used in different settings and for different purposes.

- A cassette system, in which medications are separated, organized, and stored in trays and drawers, is best for unit-dose storage of medications.
- Medication carts, which contain cassette systems for unit-dose storage, are best used in institutional settings where portability is necessary.
- Stationary wall units are best used for bulk storage of medications

Return to Manufacturer

Periodically, you may need to return drugs to the manufacturer for a variety of reasons. The most common reason drugs are returned to the manufacturer is due to expiration. **Manufacturer recalls** of a given pharmaceutical also require return. Recalls occur when there is a problem in the manufacture or distribution of a drug product that may present a risk to public health. The FDA classifies recalls in the following way:

- Class I recalls are for dangerous or defective products that could cause serious health problems or death.
- Class II recalls are for products that might cause a temporary health problem, or pose only a slight threat of a serious nature. One example of a Class II drug is a medication that is under-strength but is not used to treat life-threatening situations.
- Class III recalls are for products that are unlikely to cause any adverse health reaction, but that violate FDA labeling or manufacturing regulations.

A drug is recalled according to its lot number. When processing a manufacturer's recall notice, timely response in checking the inventory, as well as in removing affected products from the inventory, is critical to ensure public safety. In addition to recalls, you may be asked to return investigational drugs to the manufacturer for credit if they are not dispensed.

Labeling

Most states have specific requirements about what information must be included in prescription labeling, in addition to federal regulations. Prescriptions must have an affixed label before they can be dispensed to patients. This label should include:

- Date of dispensing (date of initial dispensing for Schedules III, IV, and V controlled substances) and, if given by the prescriber, therapeutic indication
- Pharmacy name and address
- Prescription identification serial number
- Name of patient
- Name of prescriber
- Directions for use and cautionary statements, if any. Directions for outpatient use should be in clear, complete sentences, use a verb (e.g. "take," "apply"), and specify dosage amount, frequency, route of administration, duration of use, and therapeutic indication.
- A federal transfer label on prescriptions for Schedule II, III, IV, and V drugs unless dispensed and administered in a healthcare facility. This label states: "Caution: Federal law prohibits the transfer of this drug to any person other than the patient for whom it was prescribed."
- A label warning against any possible adverse effects of the medication on the patient

Note that most states also require labels to contain the name and strength of the drug product dispensed. Some prescriptions require labeling beyond what will fit on the label itself. In these instances, auxiliary labels are often used to clarify or elaborate on directions for use. Auxiliary labels may include instructions such as "Shake Well" (for suspensions and emulsions) or "Take with Food" (for drugs that cause stomach upset, such as NSAIDs).

Package Inserts

In addition to auxiliary labels, some prescriptions also contain package inserts. Steroids and Accutane also require inserts. These are documents provided by the manufacturer and approved by the FDA that include additional information about medications, such as approved uses and potential side effects. Federal law requires that package inserts always be dispensed with estrogens, such as contraceptives, so that patients are aware of the risks and benefits of its use. Some drugs such as nitro bc's are exempt from the law requiring package inserts.

NDC Numbers

Drug manufacturers assign a unique numerical code to each drug they produce. This is called the **National Drug Code (NDC)**. It is an 11-digit, 3-segment number.

- The first five digits comprise the labeler code, and are assigned by the FDA. A labeler is any company that manufactures or distributes the drug.
- The next four digits are the product code, which identifies the medication, its strength, and its dosage form.
- The last two digits indicate the package size.

Controlled Substances

Controlled substances are subject to heavier regulation by federal and state laws than are over-the-counter medications. For example, pharmacies must conduct an official inventory of controlled substances once every two years. In addition to this official inventory, some pharmacies use a **perpetual inventory** method to manage the stock of controlled substances on a continuous basis. This means that each time a controlled substance is received or dispensed, it is recorded in a computerized system.

Controlled substances may be stored in a locked cabinet, dispersed throughout the inventory of non-controlled drugs, or a combination of both.

DEA Form 222

Among drugs with medical use, Schedule II drugs have the highest potential for abuse. As a result, they require a special form to be ordered from a wholesaler or supplier: DEA Form 222. DEA Form 222 contains three copies. Copies 1 and 2 are sent to the supplier or wholesaler fulfilling the order. The supplier, in turn, sends one of their two copies to the DEA. Copy 3 is retained by the pharmacy. Under DEA Form 222, CII drugs may also be ordered within the computerized DEA system.

Over-the-counter drugs

In addition to properly managing the inventory of prescription drugs, including controlled substances, you may also have important responsibilities in managing the stock of over-the-counter drugs. These include:

- Conducting inventory of over-the-counter drugs
- Removing expired drugs from the shelves
- Ordering and replenishing the stock of drugs as needed
- Returning or salvaging expired drugs

When stocking shelves with over-the-counter drugs, keep in mind that newly acquired products will generally have a longer shelf life and should be placed behind packages that will expire before them. This method is known as stock rotation or "FIFO," meaning "first in, first out."

Chapter Summary

- Inventory at a pharmacy involves conducting a physical count of all medications in possession. Par levels are predetermined quantities of medications that should be kept in stock. A list of preferred drug products should be maintained in a computerized formulary.
- Invoices for purchases should be kept by the pharmacy to document the receipt of drug orders. A pharmacy's inventory level may need adjustments on a short-term or long-term basis, depending on various factors.
- Most medications should be stored at room temperature. Cassette systems, medication carts, and stationary wall units are different storage options for pharmaceutical products.

- Federal and state laws mandate specific requirements for the labeling of prescription medications. The National Drug Code (NDC) is a 11-digit, 3-segment number assigned by manufacturers to the each drug they produce.
- The perpetual inventory method is used to track controlled substances in a pharmacy. DEA Form 222 must be used to order Schedule II drugs from a wholesaler or supplier.

The stock rotation method is used to manage inventory of over-the-counter drugs.

PRACTICE TEST QUESTIONS

Inventory Management and Handling and Storage of Medications

1. Prescriptions come into the pharmacy in a variety of ways. The most common is by:
   a. walk-ins.
   b. physician's phone in.
   c. fax.
   d. none of the above.

2. Which of the following medications must have a federal "transfer warning" label unless they are dispensed and administered by a healthcare facility?
   a. Schedule II drugs
   b. Schedule III drugs
   c. Schedule IV drugs
   d. all of the above

3. How often must a pharmacy perform a controlled substance inventory?
   a. yearly
   b. every two years
   c. every three years
   d. monthly

4. Which medication dispensing unit is excellent for bulk storage, but not for unit-dose storage?
   a. cassette systems
   b. medication carts
   c. stationary wall units
   d. floor stock

5. A technicians' duty with regard to over-the-counter drugs typically include(s):
   a. stocking.
   b. taking inventory.
   c. removing expired drugs from the shelves.
   d. all of the above.

6. The most common reason drugs are returned to the manufacturer is because:
   a. they are recalled.
   b. they are expired.

c. the wrong product is ordered.
d. they are mislabeled.

7. Which of the following methods of maintaining a formulary is the most convenient and yields the most current product information in a purchasing and inventory system?
   a. computerized formulary
   b. formulary log book
   c. want book
   d. log book

8. When documenting the receipt of pharmaceuticals for which the purchase order or manufacturer's invoice cannot be located, which of the following information should be recorded?
   a. product name and amount
   b. product name, strength, and amount
   c. date of receipt, name of receiver, product name, strength, dosage form, and amount
   d. name of wholesaler, product name, strength, dosage form, and amount

9. When controlled substances are stored in a pharmacy, where may they be kept?
   a. in a locked cabinet
   b. dispersed throughout the inventory of non-controlled drugs
   c. in a separate locked room
   d. either a or b

10. Formularies are typically updated every:
    a. 4–6 months.
    b. 12–18 months.
    c. 18–24 months.
    d. 3–4 years.

11. The type of inventory method used for controlled substances is called:
    a. stock rotation inventory.
    b. controlled inventory.
    c. perpetual inventory.
    d. closed inventory.

12. Which type of drugs can be returned to the manufacturer for credit?

    a. investigational
    b. controlled substances
    c. chemicals
    d. bulk

13. When the quantity of a pharmaceutical product in stock reaches a predetermined point, it is called a(n):

    a. stock level.
    b. par level.
    c. maximum level.
    d. ideal level.

14. The most important consideration in processing a manufacturer's recall notice is:

    a. timely response in checking the inventory.
    b. timely response in removing affected products from the inventory.
    c. receiving proper credit from the manufacturer.
    d. both a and b.

15. Which of the following statements about prescription labeling is false?

    a. Some prescriptions require labeling beyond what will fit on the label itself.
    b. Auxiliary labels are often used to clarify or elaborate on directions for use.
    c. If the patient is in a hurry, it is acceptable to dispense the prescription without an affixed label as long as the pharmacist talks to the patient about how to use the medication and he/she understands the directions.
    d. Most states have specific requirements about what information must be include in prescription labeling.

16. Temperature is very important for the storage of medication. Room temperature is considered to be:

    a. 15° to 30° C or 59° to 86°F.
    b. 2° to 8°C or 36° to 46°F.
    c. 30° to 40°C or 86° to 104°F.
    d. Above 40°C or 104°F.

17. Which of the following best incorporates all recommended components of label directions for outpatient use?

    a. Take one tablet three times daily.
    b. Take one tablet by mouth three times daily for 10 days for infection.
    c. Take one tablet by mouth three times daily for 10 days.
    d. Take one tablet three times daily for pain.

18. A situation that might require adjustment of the pharmacy's inventory level on a short-term basis is:

    a. an increased need for seasonal products, such as asthma medication.
    b. a particular patient requiring high doses of a pain medication.
    c. an extended period of high use of a particular product by multiple patients.
    d. a and b.

19. The NDC number is assigned by the manufacturer for each drug it produces. What do the individual digits in the NDC number mean?

    a. The first five digits indicate the manufacturer, the next four indicate the medication, its strength, and dosage form, and the last two digits indicate the package size.
    b. The first five digits indicate the medication, its strength, and dosage form, the next four indicate the package size, and the last two indicate the manufacturer.
    c. The first five digits indicate the manufacturer, the next four indicate the package size, and the last two indicate the medication, its strength, and dosage form.
    d. The first five digits indicate the medication, its strength, and dosage form, the next four indicate the manufacturer, and the last two indicate the package size.

20. A package insert is always dispensed to the patient for which type of medication?

    a. high blood pressure
    b. estrogens
    c. diabetic
    d. psychotropic

21. Newly acquired products will generally have a longer shelf life and should be placed behind packages that will expire before them. This procedure is called:

    a. overstocking.
    b. inventory rotation.
    c. stock rotation.
    d. perpetual inventory process.

22. The Occupational Safety and Health Administration (OSHA) requires pharmacies to have this on hand for each hazardous chemical they use:

    a. Material Safety Data Sheets
    b. United States Pharmacopoeia Drug Information
    c. Pharmacy Law Digest
    d. Facts and Comparisons

23. Inventory control may include:

   a. maintaining minimum and maximum reorder points.

   b. returning outdated stock.

   c. recording the receipt of controlled substances.

   d. all of the above.

24. The form used to order Schedule II drugs from a wholesaler or supplier is called:

   a. DEA form 203.

   b. DEA form 222.

   c. DEA form 124.

   d. DEA form 320.

25. The DEA form consists of how many parts?

   a. Two parts; the pharmacy keeps one part and returns the second one to the wholesaler.

   b. Four parts; the pharmacy keeps one part, returns the second one to the wholesaler, and the remaining two go to the DEA.

   c. One part, which stays with the pharmacy as the wholesaler already has a duplicate copy.

   d. Three parts; the pharmacy keeps one part, two are returned to the wholesaler with one copy being sent to DEA.

PART 3

Participating in the Administration and Management of Pharmacy Practice

CHAPTER 12 / Administrative Duties and Technology

CHAPTER 13 / Business Management

CHAPTER 14 / Professionalism and Personnel Management

CHAPTER 15 / Infection Control and Hazardous Materials

CHAPTER 16 / Facility Management

12

Administrative Duties and Technology

Test Topics

After completing this chapter, you should be able to demonstrate knowledge of the following:

1. Written, oral, and electronic communication systems
2. Technology used in the preparation, delivery, and administration of medications
3. Manual and computer-based systems for storing, retrieving, and using pharmacy-related information
4. Security procedures related to data integrity, security, and confidentiality
5. Backup and archiving procedures for stored data and documentation
6. Third-party reimbursement systems
7. Health care reimbursement systems
8. Billing and accounting policies and procedures
9. Information sources used to obtain data in a quality improvement system
10. Procedures to document occurrences such as medication errors, adverse effects, and product integrity

Test Terms

- **automated dispensing systems** storage, dispensing, and charging devices for medications
- **bar codes** unique arrangements of lines used to identify the item on which they are printed
- **biometric access** authentication technique that relies on measurable physical characteristics (such as a fingerprint) that can be automatically checked
- **capitation** the annual fee paid to a physician or group of physicians by each participant in a health plan
- **continuous quality improvement** a scientific and systematic process of monitoring, evaluating, and identifying problems and then developing and measuring the impact of the improvement strategies
- **fee-for-service** an insurance plan in which the patient pays out of pocket for services and then submits for reimbursement separately from the insurance plan
- **flexible spending account** a pretax-funded account that allows an employee to set aside a portion of his or her earnings to pay for qualified medical expenses
- **paraprofessional** a person who is trained to assist professionals but is not licensed at a professional level
- **risk level** the potential risk to patients caused by the introduction of microbial contamination into a finished sterile product
- **third-party billing** billing a patient's insurance company for products and services
- **unit-dose system** a packaging system in which medication is dispensed in a single dose package that is ready to administer to the patient

Outside of assisting in the preparation of prescriptions, the list of additional tasks a pharmacy technician may attend varies widely, from data entry, to restocking and ordering supplies, to filing and archiving hard copies of prescriptions. Although these tasks may be administrative in nature, they are no less important or vital to keeping a pharmacy running smoothly. Without a reliable system of checks and balances, a pharmacy could quickly spiral into chaos, and errors would undoubtedly occur.

Making these administrative tasks run more smoothly has largely been the result of an increase in the use of technology. Technology, specifically the use of computers, has advanced the practice of pharmacy by leaps and bounds just over the last 15 years. As computers have become faster, more secure, and easier to use, pharmacies have adapted their practices to rely heavily on computer technology for processing, filling, storing, and securing prescriptions. Nearly every aspect of pharmacy services is controlled or monitored by computers. As a result, there are certain assurances and legal issues that surround the storage and retrieval of patient information in these computer systems.

Communication

Despite the rise in the use of technology, pharmacy technicians are required to be skilled in written and oral communication. Face-to-face interactions with patients, pharmacists, physicians, and nurses may occur on a daily basis. As the role of the pharmacy technician continues to change, it is being viewed as a **paraprofessional** position. A paraprofessional is a person who is trained to assist professionals but is not licensed at a professional level. Pharmacy technicians can be found in roles such as:

- clinical pharmacy technicians
- inventory specialists
- nuclear medication technicians

Written and Oral Communication

Interacting with professionals and patients requires tact, sensitivity, diplomacy, and patience. Pharmacists view the greatest attribute of a pharmacy technician to be their ability to communicate clearly, effectively, and compassionately. When speaking with other professionals or with patients, you must convey, through your voice and body language, that you are concerned, serious, and reliable to not only do your job but to do it professionally. Remember that the patients you interact with are there for a reason—their own health issues—which should spur you to act compassionately and kindly toward them.

Written communication is a worthwhile attribute as well. Pharmacists, doctors, and nurses are very busy and have many demands on their concentration, so relaying patient concerns, prescription questions, or other patient-related information neatly and accurately is vital to maintaining effective communication in the pharmacy.

For example, what if a nurse calls the pharmacy with a drug interaction question? If you jot down insufficient or inaccurate information, it could result in calamity. In this example, it's important that you accurately convey the nurse's name, the floor location and extension (hospital setting) or physician's office (community setting), the purpose of the call, the time of the call, the initials of the technician who answered the call, and how a response is needed.

> **RECALL TIP**
>
> Remember the ABC's of communication: always be courteous. The perception that others have of you will translate into how capable and professional they think you are at performing your job. Remember that patients in particular need compassion and patience, as they may be dealing with serious health issues.

Electronic Communication

There is hardly a pharmacy in existence today that doesn't use a computer for prescription processing, maintaining patient information, or dispensing medication. Many physicians have come to rely on computers to transmit prescription information, which has drastically cut down on the number of prescriptions filled incorrectly as a result of illegible handwriting. Computers are used in the pharmacy for such activities as:

- quality assurance
- drug information

- drug utilization evaluations
- adverse drug reaction reporting
- nonformulary drug use
- workload statistics computing

Access to a pharmacy's computer system is typically controlled by having users sign on with a user name and password. A less frequently used method is **biometric access**, which requires the user's fingerprints. Making sure to log off each time you walk away from a computer ensures that no one else can access information using your user name and password. It is equally important that you are wary when opening and reading e-mail messages that could introduce a virus into the pharmacy's computer system. A virus can disable a system in minutes and can jeopardize patient information.

Typically, a patient's profile will contain only certain elements that are stored in a database. These profiles are particularly useful in **unit-dose systems**, which provide a 12- to 24-hour dose of medication and maintain real-time patient information. These include:

- demographic information (name, age, address, phone number, gender)
- allergies
- weight
- height
- diagnosis
- scheduled medications
- nonscheduled/nonrecurring medications
- floorstock/wardstock medication
- insurance information

In a hospital setting, this information can be used as part of patient-monitoring functions that check for:

- therapeutic duplication
- drug-allergy, drug-food, drug-disease, and drug-lab interactions
- IV compatibility

Preparation of Prescriptions

Technology has increased the speed and accuracy of preparing medication for administration. Through the use of robotics and automation, work that was previously accomplished by pharmacists and pharmacy technicians is now being done by machines, with oversight from pharmacists. The goal of these processes is to increase quality and reduce errors in the most cost-effective way.

Bar coding

Using **bar codes**, which are unique arrangements of lines used to identify the item on which they are printed, identifies a drug's:

- name
- strength
- dosage form
- lot number
- expiration date

Bar codes are useful in both community and institutional pharmacies to save time and increase accuracy when ordering and distributing medication, returning inventory, billing and crediting patients for drugs dispensed and returned, respectively, and checking unit-dose carts. They're also helpful when health care teams are working to ensure that a patient receives the correct drug, dose, and dosage form at the correct time and via the correct route of administration. Bar-coding is one of the most commonly used systems to manage controlled substance levels in a pharmacy's stock, along with the Pyxis machine.

Automated Dispensing Systems

Bar-coding is traditionally used with unit-dose systems, but that can be a labor-intensive type of delivery system because it must be operated and stocked, which mainly involved pharmacy technicians. Many inpatient and hospital settings have taken to using **automated dispensing systems**, which are storage, dispensing, and charging devices for medications. They're favored because they save time and allow for better control and tracking of inventory. There are two types of systems:

- *Decentralized Systems*—located in the patient care unit, these systems contain floor stock medication and supplies and are designed to solve medication management problems, including narcotic diversion and poor record-keeping. They're used to dispense and return medications, record medication waste, and generate reports. Examples include the Pyxis MedStation, Omnicell Sure-Med, and McKesson Acudose-Rx.
- *Centralized Systems*—located in the central pharmacy, these systems are used to improve the manual unit-dose cart-fill process that can be tedious without help. They cannot accommodate all dosage forms, such as refrigerated medications, so some manual cart-fill still takes place. Examples include AutoMed Efficiency Pharmacy and the McKesson Robot-Rx.

Robotic Cart Fill

The McKesson Robot-Rx combines bar-code technology, a computer system, a conveyor system, and a robot to pick drugs and place them into patient medication drawers or envelopes. As a result, the cart-fill process is highly accurate. Technicians are usually responsible for all aspects of this robotic dispensing system, including packaging, stocking, inventory control, cart fill, manual fill, and troubleshooting. A disadvantage to the system is the requirement of special packaging for the dispensed medications and the expense of the Robot-Rx system itself.

Process Control Devices

Institutional pharmacies often use computerized pumps in the IV admixture area to prepare total parenteral nutrition and hyperalimentation solutions, including devices such as MicroMix and AutoMix. These pumps automatically fill the base solution and any added electrolytes and micronutrients. Other computerized pumps are used to fill batches of syringes at a time. Process control devices require the pharmacy technician to operate them and to set up the correct medication solutions and log sheets used for quality assurance.

Administrative Policies and Procedures

Inpatient and community pharmacies are structured to ensure that rules and regulations are followed so that critical errors do not occur. Just as in our government, a system of checks and balances is key to maintaining workflow, quality assurance, and integrity in the pharmacy setting.

Organizational Structure

RECALL TIP

Wondering where to go with a question or problem that can't be solved by your pharmacist? Direct your queries to the Pharmacy Director. Remember that the director oversees all aspects of pharmacy operations and the intermingling of the pharmacy department with other parts of the institution.

In order to maintain quality and responsibility, there must be levels of accountability within an inpatient or community pharmacy. Without clear levels of management and a definitive chain of command, the activities of employees would become unproductive and inefficient. Inpatient or hospital pharmacies have a greater amount of oversight and chain of command than community pharmacies.

The pharmacy director is at the top of the pharmacy department hierarchy. Depending on the size of the hospital, the director may have several levels of management beneath them. Because they are beholden to the hospital for their funding and location, the pharmacy director reports to a hospital administrator. Pharmacy directors are responsible for the activity and materials management within the pharmacy, but they do not operate separately from the other departments in the hospital. The pharmacy works in tandem with many departments, including billing and patient records, to meet patient needs and ascertain critical information.

Billing and Accounting

Transmitting information to insurance companies is another task of the pharmacy technician. It involves the knowledge of formulary and nonformulary drugs, generic and trade names, types of insurance plans, and limitations based on the length of a medication's supply.

Third-Party Billing

Third-party billing refers to the third part of the three parties involved in the payment process: patient, pharmacy, and insurance company. Once a patient has paid their portion of the drug cost which is either a flat rate (copay), variable rate, or a straight percentage, the remainder is submitted to an insurance company for reimbursement. There are four types of insurance plans:

- *Health maintenance organizations* (HMOs)—patient chooses a primary care physician, receives a discounted rate for attending a contracted provider, pays an annual fee for participation in the insurance (known as **capitation**), and pays a predetermined amount for services, known as the copay.

- *Preferred provider organization* (PPO)—patient may visit any doctor without choosing a primary care physician, usually pays higher out-of-pocket expenses than an HMO patient, and pays a copay for services rendered and any costs beyond the coverage of the insurance plan. A subtype of PPO is a **fee-for-service** plan, where the patient pays out of pocket for services and then submits for reimbursement separately from the insurance plan.

- *Government programs* (Medicare and Medicaid)—patients are senior citizens, disabled, or are receiving dialysis (Medicare) or are low-income (Medicaid); pay a deductible and a percentage of the cost of services provided (Medicare); and may or may not receive prescription drug benefits.

- *Worker's compensation*—insurance extended by an employer to employees who have been injured on the job; patients do not pay any out-of-pocket costs.

RECALL TIP

One way to distinguish between Medicare and Medicaid recipients is to remember that Medicare recipients are typically seniors being cared for, while Medicaid recipients are receiving financial aid.

Insurance companies require the following information in order to process a claim for reimbursement:

- patient's name
- date of medication fill
- pharmacy name and address
- medication prescribed
- dosage

- patient's date of birth
- insurance identification number

Health Care Reimbursement

In a health care reimbursement plan, often known as a **flexible spending account (FSA)**, participants make pre-tax contributions by payroll deduction, and the funds are maintained by a third party commissioned by the patient's employer. The patient can submit for reimbursement of covered expenses, such as:

- copays
- deductibles
- orthodontic care
- over-the-counter non-prescription drugs
- vision and hearing expenses
- home health care expenses not covered by an insurance plan

You may be asked to provide a detailed receipt for an over-the-counter medication for a patient to submit to their provider.

> **RECALL TIP**
>
> FSAs and they types of costs they reimburse are mostly universal, but some plans reimburse for expenses other than drug and medical, such as daycare. One way to remind patients to use their FSA dollars is that FSA also stands for Funds Stay Away – if they don't use their monies, they lose them at the end of the calendar year.

Quality Assurance and Legal Measures

There are several governing bodies that oversee the licensing, policies, and procedures of pharmacies and pharmacists. Each state has its own Board of Pharmacy, and they license pharmacists and monitor that pharmacies are maintaining certain requirements. Despite great interest in pharmacy technician certification programs by students and pharmacists alike, there are currently no federal requirements for their training and licensing. Some individual states have established requirements, and more information is available through each state's Board of Pharmacy.

Pharmacy laws are designed to protect patients and the public in general from danger or negligence. Pharmacy law ensures that:

- A knowledgeable individual double-checks the results of the prescribing process and oversees the use of medications
- A licensed pharmacist is on duty whenever the pharmacy is open
- Licensed pharmacists graduate from an accredited school of pharmacy, pass a licensure examination, and pass the state's board examination.

> **RECALL TIP**
>
> Medication errors in the pharmacy can be deadly, so remember CDC: check-double-check your drug pulls, labels, and calculations. You never know when mistakes can happen.

The Technician's Role

Despite the fact that pharmacy technicians have taken on increasing responsibilities in pharmacies, they are still support staff to the pharmacists. In some states, they do not hold a license and therefore cannot dispense medication without the supervision of a licensed pharmacist. Most states, however, do require technicians to have a license to practice. For the most part, technicians can only make nonjudgmental discussions. In addition, because they have not received the schooling and preparation in the field of clinical pharmacy, they are not allowed to counsel patients on their medication. More and more patients require counseling, which is why clinical pharmacy practices have penetrated every aspect of both inpatient and community pharmacy. In a world where physicians spend increasingly less time with their patients, pharmacists are required to counsel patients on potential drug interactions and monitor the use and administration of medications that may or may not have been dispensed by them. That is why it is imperative that as a pharmacy technician, you never counsel patients on their medication, regardless of how minor the question or how busy the pharmacist; errant advice could lead to drastic consequences.

What are some ways a technician ensures quality and integrity in the pharmacy? Being alert to suspicious prescriptions is a very important way. You can help the pharmacist flag a potential forgery or abuse situation by watching for prescriptions that are:

- written for a large quantity of a controlled substance
- missing a DEA number for a scheduled drug
- illegible and could be written for any number of similarly named drugs
- written by an unfamiliar or out-of-town physician

You are the first eyes on the prescription, so it is important that you stay alert. It is your job to bring to the pharmacist's attention anything out of the ordinary.

Continuous Quality Improvement

Continuous quality improvement (CQI) is a scientific and systematic process of monitoring, evaluating, and identifying problems and then developing and measuring the impact of the improvement strategies. The focus of CQI is on the problems within a system, not on people or patients. Everyone who is part of the pharmacy department should participate in CQI brainstorming and evaluations that are designed to improve the problems identified. In fact, many accrediting agencies, such as the Joint Commission on the Accreditation of Healthcare Organizations (JCAHO) require pharmacies to participate in quality control and quality improvement programs. You as a pharmacy technician are invaluable in preparing surveys or inspections by these governing agencies.

Quality Assurance

Whether you're providing clinical or product-focused services to patients, the focus should always be on doing so with the greatest emphasis on quality. Medication quality and safety continues to be spotlighted by the JCAHO and other accrediting and regulatory agencies, as it should be. "Quality" isn't necessarily a measurable entity. It can:

- designate when a product meets certain standards
- be the positive perception of a product by customers
- embody a system of checks and balances
- refer to the level of sterility that is required for certain preparations

Quality Control

It is only recently that a set of enforceable universal precautions has been widely available and accepted. This standard, issued by the United States Pharmacopeia (USP), is *USP Chapter 797*, and it provides the procedures and requirements for compounding sterile preparations. These precautions are determined so that compounding and other pharmacy preparations may be done in the most sterile environment possible, lowering the risk of contamination. As a pharmacy technician, your tasks may require you to work in a clean room environment to ensure the sterility of the products you are preparing. Any environment that requires this level of assurance will provide written procedures and training for all employees, and checks and balances occur at critical points in the process.

Quality control prevents defective products from reaching patients, and it is particularly crucial when intravenous (IV) products are being prepared. An error or defect in an IV product may lead to illness and even death.

Risk Levels

The USP provides clear guidelines regarding the **risk levels** associated with preparing sterile products. There are four specific categories:

- immediate-use products
- low-risk products
- medium-risk products
- high-risk products

The risk levels are assigned based on the likelihood that a product will be contaminated by microbes or by chemical or physical matter. As a technician, these levels will come into play for the most part when preparing IV solutions. Generally, the less sterile the environment and the greater the number of interactions with nonsterile or potentially contaminated items, the higher the risk level. For example, immediate-use products are used within 1 hour of preparation, such as in an emergency department. On the other hand, a high-risk level product might be one which is prepared in a nonsterile device or environment, such as and IV preparation in a home health care setting.

RECALL TIP

The risk levels of contamination increase from low to high risk based on the amount of potential contamination that a sterile product may come across as it is being prepared. You may see these risk levels as either levels 1, 2, and 3, or as low, medium, and high. Remember that the higher the number, the greater number of contaminants have been introduced into the sterile preparation environment.

Medication Errors

Every instance of medication error is cause to reevaluate the standards and practices that a pharmacy has in place. The outcomes of medication errors can result in:

- no effect
- minor discomfort
- devastating long-term effects
- death

They can cause an increase in hospital stays and health care expenses, and legal fees and out-of-court settlements can result in billions of dollars spent annually. There are a number of ways that medication errors can occur:

- *Calculation errors*—including miscalculated doses and the use of the wrong strength of stock solutions
- *Decimal points and zeros*—may occur when writing orders or adding unnecessary trailing zeros, omitting the zero in front of the decimal point, or when a decimal point is hidden on lined paper
- *Abbreviations*—either in dosage units or for common drug names, such as AZT, which could be interpreted as zidovudine (antiretroviral agent) or azathioprine (an immunosuppressant)
- *High-Alert medications*—including insulin, narcotics and opiates, KCl injection, heparin, and concentrated NaCl can cause fatal reactions if given incorrectly
- *Prescribing issues*—an error in verbal orders, confusion with the concentration of a product, illegible handwriting, missing information, use of the apothecary system, and writing doses based on the course of therapy rather than on the daily dose
- *Look-alike and sound-alike drug names*—more than 750 confusing drug names (both trade and generic names) is available on the USP website

There are several ways to avoid the occurrence of medication errors. First, the JCAHO recommends that institutions maintain an approved list of acceptable abbreviations and terms. In addition, they should maintain a list of unacceptable abbreviations. Writing out the complete drug name, preferably the generic form, should eliminate confusion as well. One way to avoid calculation errors is to ask a colleague, either a pharmacist or another pharmacy technician, to check your work.

RECALL TIP

Pediatric preparation errors can be the most deadly. When receiving a prescription for a pediatric patient, think P2C2: pediatric preparations check twice! It's even better if the second check is through the eyes of a coworker.

Make it a habit to double-check your calculations especially as it pertains to pediatric preparations; the smallest error in medications prescribed for the smallest people can lead to the most profound effects.

Incident Reporting

The U.S. Food and Drug Administration (FDA) has a toll-free number for the reporting of any defect found in over-the-counter or prescription medications or any drug problems that arise. MedWatch is a voluntary reporting program that the FDA has put into effect for both consumers and health care workers to report adverse effects with medications. Things that should be reported include:

- a product that looks different from its normal package
- adverse reactions to a product
- medication reaction that causes disability, hospitalization, or death

Medication errors that occur within the pharmacy before the patient receives the medication are handled through the completion of an organization's medication error report. It is filled out and reviewed by those involved in the error, and it is forwarded onto the next level of management and the organization's quality assurance committee. Ways that a pharmacy can address medication errors include:

- publishing summaries of errors that have occurred in staff newsletters
- conducting educational programs
- discussing medication errors as part of a regular staff meeting

Medication errors are taken very seriously. Besides institutional or company liability, the pharmacist or pharmacy technician may be held accountable personally for medication error involving injury to a patient.

Security

As much as technology has improved the job of dispensing and controlling medication, it has also become a concern regarding the privacy of patient information. The concern that a patient's medical records and personal data may be compromised is a very real one, and it should be taken seriously.

Privacy

All federal, state, and common laws contain privacy laws. The violation of privacy rights by a pharmacist, technician, and pharmacy can have severe consequences. Generally, no patient information can be given to anyone other than the patient or his or her legal representative. The employer is not necessarily the patient's legal representative just because they are paying for the insurance coverage. It is unlawful to release information, without expressed consent, to a patient's:

- insurance company
- spouse
- child
- relative
- caregiver

If a request is made by telephone, it may be unwise to release information because the caller's identity cannot be identified.

Health Insurance Portability and Accountability Act of 1996 (HIPAA)

The enforcement of HIPAA has strengthened patient privacy rights. Patient records must be guarded from disclosure to anyone unauthorized to receive them, including companies and other individuals. Pharmacy employees may not discuss a patient's medical history except as it pertains to the patient's current care. Any written documentation about a patient must be discarded safely to protect their information, using shredders or a document disposal service. In a retail setting, it may be undermine a person's privacy to use the overhead paging system to call the patient to the pharmacy. Ask your institution about their policies and procedures regarding HIPAA.

Chapter Summary

- Face-to-face, written, and oral communication between pharmacy technicians and patients, professionals, and pharmacists is crucial to instilling confidence and professionalism.
- Most pharmacies use user names and passwords to protect their systems from infiltration.
- Unit-dose systems maintain real-time patient information and provide 12 to 24 hours of medication.
- Bar-coding uniquely identifies a medication's vital information and can link a patient with his or her medication.
- Automated dispensing systems are favored because they save time and allow for better tracking and control of inventory.
- Robotic cart-fills are highly accurate and useful means for filling patient medication orders.
- Pharmacy directors are responsible for the activity and materials management of a pharmacy and work in tandem with other departments in an institution.
- Pharmacy technicians use computer systems to bill insurance companies for a patient's products and services.
- Insurance plans include HMOs, PPOs, Medicare, Medicaid, and worker's compensation.
- Health care reimbursement plans (or flexible spending accounts) allow participants to put aside pretax dollars to spend on allowed medical expenses.
- Technicians are not legally allowed to counsel patients or dispense medication; only licensed pharmacists may do so.
- Being alert for suspicious prescriptions helps the pharmacist to maintain integrity in the dispensation of medication.
- Continuous quality improvement focuses on the problems within a system.
- *USP Chapter 797* provides the procedures and requirements for compounding sterile preparations and outlines the levels of contamination risk.
- Contamination risk levels include immediate-use, low risk, medium risk, and high risk.
- Medication errors effects on patients range from no effect to death, and the fiduciary responsibility of institutions and companies for such errors may be astronomical.
- The FDA uses MedWatch as a means of voluntary reporting of adverse effects or compromised medication.
- Patient information should be fiercely guarded, and by law, no patient information can be given to anyone other than the patient or his or her legal representative.

PRACTICE TEST QUESTIONS

Administrative Duties and Technology

1. Licensing and general professional oversight of pharmacists and pharmacies is carried out by:

   a. College of Pharmacy
   b. The American Pharmaceutical Society
   c. The United States Pharmacopoeia Convention
   d. State pharmacy boards

2. The purpose of the clinical pharmacy is to:

   a. dispense medications
   b. provide information about medication
   c. compound medication
   d. report adverse reaction or interactions of medication

3. At present, no federal requirements and few state requirements exist for the training and licensing of pharmacy technicians.

   a. true
   b. false

4. A person who assists professionals in carrying out their duties is called a:

   a. druggist
   b. toxicologist
   c. paraprofessional
   d. none of the above

5. A technician carries out many of the same duties as a pharmacist and depending on the facility can dispense medication without the supervision of a pharmacist.

   a. true
   b. false

6. Of the automated systems listed, which is the most commonly used to manage controlled substances levels?

   a. Pyxis machine
   b. Baker Cell System
   c. Bar coding
   d. both a and c

7. A set of standards used to prepare medications that lower the possibility of contamination is:

   a. universal precautions
   b. aseptic technique
   c. guidelines for handwashing
   d. guidelines for hood cleaning

8. In a hospital, the overall responsibility for the materials management of pharmaceuticals lies with the:

   a. Chairman of the Pharmacy and Therapeutics Committee
   b. Hospital Board of Directors
   c. Director of Pharmacy Services
   d. Materials Manager

9. When a filling label seems to indicate an error, which of the following would be an appropriate initial action for the technician?

   a. alert the pharmacist that an error has been made
   b. check the label against the original order to determine if an error was made
   c. call the physician to clarify the order
   d. call the nursing unit (institutional setting) or notify the patient (outpatient setting) that an error was made on the prescription order

10. Besides choosing the correct drug entity, which of the following decisions must be made at the time an IV drug is being chosen during a computerized order entry process in the hospital?

    a. the correct dosage for the amount being prepared
    b. the correct dosage form for the route of administration
    c. the correct dilute solution
    d. all of the above

11. An example of the automation machines used to prepare hyperalimentation solutions is/are:

    a. Robot-Rx
    b. MicroMix and AutoMix
    c. SureMed
    d. none of the above

12. Which of the following statements regarding quality is *false*?

    a. quality control is a process of checks and balances
    b. quality may be defined by what customers perceive
    c. because quality is something that cannot be directly measured, it is more important to focus on the quantity of products made
    d. quality is determined by the cleanliness of the pharmacy

13. Which of the following is *not* true of hospital pharmacy dispensing automation?

    a. both centralized and decentralized automation make dispensing more efficient
    b. decentralized automation is superior to centralized automation
    c. some institutions combine both centralized and decentralized automation to incorporate advantages of both systems
    d. dispensing automation may be centralized in the pharmacy or decentralized at the point of care

14. Any suspicious prescription should be brought to the attention of the pharmacist because it may be a forgery.

    a. true
    b. false

15. Which of the following statements regarding pharmacy directors is *false*?

    a. pharmacy directors often report to one of the hospital's administrators
    b. pharmacy directors are at the top of the pharmacy department's personnel
    c. pharmacy directors are responsible for the activity within the pharmacy
    d. pharmacy directors can operate all activities independent of other departments or managers

16. A pharmacy technician is preparing a 1-week supply of total parenteral nutrition for a patient at home using an automated compounding device. Investigational L-glutamine is being added at the end of the mixing process. Which risk level of compounding describes this situation?

    a. Immediate-use
    b. Low-risk
    c. Medium-risk
    d. High-risk

17. A flexible spending account requires:

    a. the employee to pay a co-pay for their provider services
    b. the employer to set aside a portion of an employees earning for qualified expenses
    c. the physician to pay an annual fee to participate in the insurance plan
    d. the patient to pay out-of-pocket for services and then submits a receipt to the insurance plan for reimbursement

18. Which of the following statements about CQI is/are *false*?

    a. CQI focuses on people problems
    b. CQI allows decisions to be made on the basis of objective data alone
    c. CQI is a scientific/systematic approach to quality
    d. a & b

19. What are the two major mechanisms for third-party pharmacy reimbursement?

    a. POS and fee-for-service
    b. capitation and POS

    c. copayments and deductibles
    d. fee-for-service and capitation

20. Which of the following is *not* a copayment arrangement designated by third parties?

    a. fee-for-service
    b. flat rate
    c. variable rate
    d. straight percentage

21. Communication skills and customer service are the most important qualifications of a pharmacy technician. Which duty is *not* a responsibility of a technician?

    a. handle demanding patients appropriately
    b. counseling patients on their medication
    c. computer order entry
    d. prescription filling and labeling

22. Access to the pharmacy computer system is controlled by:

    a. finger print touch screen
    b. signature of the pharmacy personnel
    c. user name and password
    d. combination of finger print and signature

23. Current computer technology used in health care today is:

    a. bar coding
    b. touch screens
    c. automated dispensing systems
    d. all of the above

24. Information needed on the patient's medication profile includes all the following *except*:

    a. whether the patient is married or single
    b. dosage strength and form
    c. insurance provider
    d. duration time of medication

25. Which of the following statements is a disadvantage of the robotic cart fill system?

    a. the use of bar coding provides accuracy in identify the patient
    b. good inventory control
    c. special packaging and equipment for the system
    d. removal of expired drugs before they are dispensed

13

Business Management

Test Topics

After completing this chapter, you should be able to demonstrate knowledge of the following:

1. The practice setting's mission, goals and objectives, organizational structure, and policies and procedures.
2. Productivity, efficiency and customer satisfaction measures.

Test Terms

- **community pharmacists** stand-alone businesses that fill prescriptions as well as nonprescription products for ambulatory patients
- **home health pharmacy** pharmacies that are based away from hospital sites and not open to the public, couriers deliver the medications to the home health clients
- **inpatient pharmacy** pharmacy located in a hospital where patients stay overnight or longer; have a wider range of stock than outpatient pharmacies because they provide the specific medication and supplies for every department in the hospital
- **mail-order pharmacy** large distribution pharmacies that dispense medication through the mail
- **managed care pharmacy** operate much like a community or other ambulatory care pharmacies, but carry only drugs that are on the organization's formulary and serve only patients covered on their plan
- **outpatient pharmacy** a pharmacy that is not connected with a hospital
- **pharmaceutical business** merges the fields of healthcare and business, combining the key elements of pharmaceutical-science and pharmaceutical-marketing programs
- **pharmaceutical companies** specialize in the research, development, and marketing of medicines
- **pharmaceuticals manufacturers** take raw materials and process them into finished medicines ready for the consumer
- **policy** a high-level, overall plan, and a definite course or method of action selected from among alternatives
- **procedure** a traditional or standard way of doing things
- **third-party programs** insurance or entitlement programs that reimburse the pharmacy for products delivered and services rendered

The pharmacy is responsible for assuring that patients receive the proper drug therapy for their specific medical needs. To achieve this goal, pharmacy personnel perform a variety of duties designed to deliver consistently the correct drug in the correct amount to all patients. These duties range from ordering medications from suppliers to distributing drugs to patients. Pharmacists are assisted by pharmacy technicians to fulfill these obligations.

Pharmaceutical business merges the fields of healthcare and business. It combines the key elements of pharmaceutical science and pharmaceutical marketing. According to the U.S. Department of Labor and Statistics, careers in pharmaceutical and biotechnology industries are expected to far exceed growth in other industries, leaving major pharmaceutical businesses in an excellent position for continued expansion.

Pharmaceutical companies specialize in the research, development, and marketing of medicines. The market for these medicines is growing, reflecting an increased demand for healthcare. As a result, pharmaceutical manufacturing operates in a rapidly changing high technology environment.

Organizational Structure and Corporate Services

Healthcare institutions are typically organized into several levels of management. Managers at the top of an organization are primarily involved in setting a direction and vision for the hospital. The organizational structure is important because it enhances communication, teamwork, and decision-making within the healthcare institution. It also outlines the formal authority and communication networks within individual departments. Each employee is encouraged to use this organizational structure to verify that communications, suggestions and/or problems are directed to the individual directly responsible for that area. Any issues that cannot be resolved by an employee's direct supervisor are directed to the next highest level in the organizational structure.

A pharmaceutical department may be organized, for example, in service-practice areas (e.g., Inpatient Operations, Ambulatory Operations, Business Services, and so on), each of which would be managed by an individual at the Director level. The Directors would report to the Administrator of Pharmaceutical Services, who in turn would reports to the Associate Hospital Director for Professional Services. Continuing with this example, the Pharmaceutical Services Department would be managed by the Director of Pharmacy, who would report to the Director of Operations. The Director of Operations would report to the Chief Operating Officer.

Some pharmacy services are more effectively provided via a corporate services delivery model. This means that the services are offered from a centralized location to more than one facility in an organization. The following are examples of pharmacy corporate services:

- Ambulatory Clinic
- Billing
- Chemotherapy Management
- Financial Management
- Investigational Drug
- Pharmacy Informatics
- Policy and Compliance
- Procurement
- Technician Program

> **RECALL TIP**
>
> Director of Operations and Chief Operating Officer seem like similar titles. In order to remember who reports to who, think of the alphabet. C comes before D, so the <u>C</u>hief Operating Officer has more power. The <u>D</u>irector of Operations should report to him or her.

Pharmacy Policies and Procedures

Every pharmacy has a binder of standard policies and procedures. A **policy** is a high-level, overall plan, and a definite course or method of action selected from among alternatives. A **procedure** is a traditional or standard way of doing things.

These policies and procedures pertain to medications, inventory, order of operations, work schedules, and specific skills and/or tasks required of pharmacy staff. Pharmacy staff can also find in this binder policies pertaining to job duties and employee benefits, as well as job orientation, training and evaluation methods. These policies are developed by the pharmacy's management and are updated regularly. The binder also outlines procedures for error reporting, discrepancies, and other areas of concern. Every pharmacy technician should become acquainted with the binder of policies and procedures.

It is necessary that all legal and professional requirements are observed in every pharmacy. All appropriate policies and procedures must be established, maintained and reviewed. The pharmacy owner, superintendent pharmacist or pharmacy manager in a hospital has overall responsibility for setting out the standards and policies for the provision of pharmacy services by the organization. The pharmacist (or pharmacy technician with management responsibilities) must ensure that policies and procedures are appropriate for the particular department or premises he or she is responsible for. He or she must guarantee that:

- Policies and standard operating procedures for safety and effective provision of pharmacy services in accordance with relevant legal and professional requirements are in place, maintained and regularly reviewed.
- Clear lines of accountability exist and a retrievable audit trail of the health professional taking responsibility for the provision of each pharmacy service is maintained.
- Appropriate policies for the number and required experience levels of staff for the business or department(s) are in place and made known to relevant staff.
- Suitable arrangements are in place when members of staff are off duty and effective handover procedures are followed.
- There are systems to identify and manage risks to patients, the public, and employees themselves. There must be procedures to deal with incidents that pose a threat to the safety of the patient, public, and employee. It is important to review practices in light of such incidents.
- Procedures are in place to record errors or minor accidents, notify the person responsible, and review procedures as appropriate.
- Procedures respect and protect confidential information about patients and employees in accordance with current legislation, relevant codes of practice, and professional guidelines.
- Systems are in place to ensure that the supplier and the quality of any medicines, devices, and pharmaceutical ingredients obtained are reputable.
- Appropriate security measures are in place to protect stocks of medicinal products, devices, and pharmaceutical ingredients, especially those which may be at particular risk of theft or abuse.
- Any advertising and promotional activities authorized for professional services or medicinal products comply with appropriate advertising codes of practice, professional guidance, and the law.

In addition to the legal requirements outlined above, the pharmacy and pharmacy technician professions have a Code of Ethics, which states seven principles of ethical practice that you must follow. The Code of Ethics demands that pharmacy staff "Take responsibility for [their] working practices" and sets out the expectations for applying this principle in practice.

Pharmaceutical Manufacturing

Pharmaceuticals manufacturers take raw materials and process them into finished medicines ready for the consumer. There are three major stages of production:

1. *Research and Development*: The R&D process can last up to 12 years from initial discovery to regulatory approval. During this time, thousands of compounds are screened to determine if they can be used in a new medicine. They are then tested and tried before they are manufactured.

2. *Primary Manufacture*: In the primary manufacturing stage, raw materials are combined and processed to make the active ingredient that goes into a medicine. This can involve a simple mixing or more complex chemical reactions.

3. *Secondary Manufacture*: In the secondary manufacturing stage, the active ingredient is turned into a medicine by mixing it with other substances to produce tablets that are the appropriate size, texture and taste. These other substances are called excipients and they make up most of the volume of the medicine

Regulation and Quality Assurance

The systems and equipment used in the manufacture and sale of medicines are highly regulated by the government and need to be validated before a manufacturing license can be granted. In order to validate its equipment, the company must demonstrate that the system and equipment consistently produce a product of the required quality.

Human Resources

The pharmaceutical business is an industry in which keeping up with the quality of the medicine is absolutely vital. As a result, the people that the companies employ are a key source. Employees are needed to staff the following departments:

- Quality Operation—involves testing raw materials and finished goods
- Primary Production—includes fermentation, organics, drying, milling and blending
- Secondary Production—involves manufacturing and packaging of medicines
- Engineering—includes repair and maintenance, project engineering, utilities and waste management

Pharmacy Settings and Productivity

In the 1990s and again in 2009-2010, healthcare reform became a major item on political agendas. With respect to pharmacies, there has been a great deal of debate about the cost of pharmaceuticals. Attempts to manage the cost of pharmacy services and products resulted in the expansion of managed care and mail-order pharmacy operations and the advent of pharmacy benefit management firms (PBMs).

There are Several Different Types of Pharmacies:

- An **inpatient pharmacy** is one that is located in hospitals in which patients stay overnight or longer. They have wider range of stock than outpatient pharmacies, because they provide the specific medication and supplies for every department in the hospital.

- The **outpatient pharmacy** is a pharmacy that is not connected with a hospital. Pharmacy technicians in outpatient pharmacies have a lot of front-line interaction with patients, so they must have excellent communication skills.

- A **home health pharmacy** prepares the drugs with the same type of labeling required for patient use as inpatient or outpatient pharmacies. Most home health pharmacies are based away from hospital sites and not open to the public. Couriers deliver the medications to the home health clients.

- The **mail–order pharmacy** and e-pharmacy, which allow patients to order and receive their medication via mail, are growing as the "baby boomer" generation ages. The need to fill prescriptions increases with more medications becoming available to treat commonly acquired illnesses specific to older persons. Large distribution centers process new prescriptions and refills. By using mail order, patients normally receive drugs at lesser cost. The role of the technicians in these pharmacies is usually the same as in other ambulatory care sites, except the technician has no face-to-face patient contact. Instead, most communication with patients occurs over the telephone.

Overlapping with the pharmacy settings described above are community and chain pharmacies, ambulatory pharmacies, managed-care pharmacies, and clinical pharmacies.

Community and Chain Pharmacies

Community pharmacies are often stand-alone businesses that fill prescriptions and sell a variety of nonprescription products (e.g., cough and cold preparations, toiletries). Most community pharmacies employ pharmacists and pharmacy technicians, and the pharmacist often counsel patients about proper uses of their medication.

Independent pharmacies are likely to be recognized as the "corner drug store." Their services vary, depending on the pharmacist, location, and patient population served. The owner of most independent pharmacies is the pharmacist-in-charge. Many independent pharmacies specialize in such areas as durable medical equipment (DME) or medical supplies and compounding. Some independent pharmacies also serve nursing homes.

A corporate-owned group of companies is generally recognized as a chain pharmacy. These pharmacies are usually large business entities with common policies and procedures (e.g. CVS, Walgreens). Pharmacies as well as technicians are employees of the corporation. Chain pharmacies often offer discount prescription-filling services, accept a large number of insurance plans, and offer the convenience of multiple locations. Some chains (as well as some independent pharmacies) also offer cholesterol screening, flu shots, and blood pressure monitoring services.

Ambulatory Care

Ambulatory care is all health-related services for patients who walk to seek their care. Examples are: clinics, emergency rooms, private offices, and community pharmacies. Traditionally, the ambulatory care practice site has been the community pharmacy.

The type of information ambulatory care pharmacies manage is similar to the type inpatient pharmacies manage (e.g., patient drug profile, inventory management). An important distinction between ambulatory care pharmacies and institutional pharmacies is that ambulatory care pharmacies are responsible for billing and collecting payments for their products, whereas institutional pharmacies may be responsible for billing, but not collecting payment. Ambulatory care pharmacists need payer and insurance carrier information and third-party billing functions as part of the computer database.

Ambulatory pharmacy computer functions fall under three main categories:

- Database maintenance
- Interfaces with other systems
- Management functions

Database maintenance tends to include tasks such as maintaining drug files, physician files, and payer and insurance information. When interfacing with other systems, the

RECALL TIP

Remember that the word "ambulatory" comes from "to ambulate," which means to move from place to place, or more simply, to walk. Thus, ambulatory care is for those who are able to walk, or ambulate, in order to seek care.

computers are able to access patient information, information on prescription processing, pharmacist authorizations, and price inquiries. Finally, the computer systems can help with certain management functions, including the generation and distribution of reports.

Managed Care Pharmacies

Managed Care Pharmacies operate much like community or other ambulatory care pharmacies but may carry only drugs on the organization's formulary and serve only the patients enrolled in the managed care plan.

Clinical Pharmacies

Clinical pharmacies and pharmacies in physician office buildings usually offer the same scope of services as many community pharmacies, but may have less focus on selling retail products other than medications. Because of the proximity of these pharmacies to the prescribers, the pharmacies generally have greater access to patient information.

Clinic pharmacies and physician office building pharmacies may differ in ownership and licensure. Clinical pharmacies associated with a hospital are likely to be owned by the hospital and operated under the direction of the hospital pharmacy department. Because of this relationship, the hospital-owned pharmacy may receive contract pricing from a buying group, through the manufacturer or through disproportionate share pricing (hospitals and clinics serving a disproportionate share of indigent patients are eligible to buy pharmaceuticals at government rates). In these instances, the pharmacists are not allowed to dispense prescriptions to nonhospital patients because their pricing gives them an unfair advantage over community pharmacies.

Filling Prescriptions

Filling prescriptions is one of the most important and commonly performed duties of a technician, regardless of the setting. Before a prescription is filled, the patient may need to consult with the pharmacist. At the time of consultation, the pharmacist also finds out which other medications the patient is taking.

There basic steps for filling a prescription are:

- *Taking and interpreting.* A prescription can be in the form of a written order that is on a prescription pad, and can be carried in to the pharmacy by hand or can be faxed from the doctor's office to the pharmacy. Prescriptions may also come in via phone, and computer-generated prescriptions are becoming more common.

- *Transcribing or translating.* When reading an order that is difficult to decipher, make sure to look at the whole order. If you are in doubt, ask another technician or the pharmacist.

- *Entering information and producing labels.* In a community setting, the technician usually enters the doctor's orders or prescription into a database or other computer system, which produces the label. The label is then checked against the prescription after its filled.

- *Filling.* After the prescription label is prepared; it is matched with the original order and is sent to the counter for filling. This may be an automated dispensing system. Again, the technician (in most settings) receives the order.

- *Checking.* When a technician take on the role of filing a patient's prescription, it is very important that he or she always remember the basic rights of a patient— to receive the correct medication in the correct dosage and amount. Checking the prescription at least three times during the filling process helps to ensure accuracy.

Managing Inventory

Technicians are typically in charge of all the aspects of ordering, restocking, and returning stock within the pharmacy. The established level of medication stock on hand at any given time is referred to as the periodic automatic replenishment level. This is the minimum amount of medication that should be maintained in the pharmacy at any given time. The drugs in a pharmacy's inventory may be loosely categorized in this way:

- *Formulary vs. non-formulary*. Non-formulary drugs are normally kept at a lower level of stock because they are not ordered often.
- *Fast mover*. These drugs typically are kept separate area from the normal stock, allowing easier access and restocking, because of the high volume of use.
- *Slow mover*. These drugs are prescribed regularly by a few doctors but are not commonly prescribed.
- *Special orders*. These typically are drugs that are used by only a few patients.
- *Seasonal*. Some drugs may be more in demand at certain times of the year.

Stock may arrive daily to a pharmacy. For billing purposes, it is important that all stock be checked completely against the invoice when first received. It is also important to follow the manufacturer's requirements for storage.

With regard to formulary vs. non-formulary drugs, think of the formulary as the backbone. The formulary is a list that describes all the medications covered under insurance plans, as well as offering alternative medications if the first choice is not covered. For medications to become part of a formulary, they must meet certain requirements, such as effectiveness and cost. Formularies are not the same at all pharmacies. A pharmacy can have an "open" formulary, which means any drug can be ordered and stocked for patient use, whereas a "closed" formulary limits the drugs that are ordered and can be used by patients.

Many formulary drugs are generic. These drugs are as effective as the brand name drugs but are less expensive. A committee composed of pharmacists, physicians, and other healthcare administrator reviews drugs that have been approved by the Food and Drug Administrators (FDA) and that are cost-effective. In addition, consideration may be given to drug companies that bid or given rebates when their drug is chosen. This decrease in price to the pharmacy ultimately saves money for the insurance company and the patient. Although most insurance companies cover most of the cost of a generic drug, some allow the patient to choose the brand-name drug.

Typically, the types of drugs not included on a formulary are new drugs, uncommon drugs, and extremely expensive drugs. However, if a non-formulary drug can be justified as a medically necessary substitution by the physician, it may be approved.

Third Party Programs

Filling prescriptions is the "meat and potatoes" of the pharmacy business, but many technicians are also in charge of the billing process and must be well aware of the policies and procedures of their pharmacy and how to process various insure claims. One of the major elements of the billing process is third party programs.

Third-party programs are insurance or entitlement programs that reimburse the pharmacy for products delivered and services rendered. There are only two major mechanisms for pharmacy reimbursement: fee-for-service and capitation.

In a fee-for-service system, patients pay cash for the prescription and submit receipts to their insurance carrier directly each time an eligible product is dispensed or services rendered. The third party then reimburses the pharmacy. The amount charged and amount reimbursed depend on the cost and the time involved. For patients without insurance, this is an "out-of-pocket" expense.

Under a capitation payment program, a pharmacy receives a set amount of money for a defined group of patients, regardless of the number of prescriptions or amount of services rendered. The dollar amount is usually in terms of per patient (member) per month.

Many third party systems require the patient to pay a copayment or meet a deductible each time a prescription is received. Third parties designate three basic copayment arrangements: (1) flat rate, (2) variable rate, and (3) straight percentage. A flat rate requires specific copay regardless of the drug received and its cost. A variable-rate copay changes depending on the product being dispensed. In perhaps its simplest form, the variable-rate copay is the multitier copay, which may be low for a generic, mid-level for a brand product on formulary, and high for a brand name off formulary.

Many pharmacists accept a large number of insurance plans, and the technicians should be familiar with the requirements of each plan or at least know where to find the information. The laws and regulations regarding generic substitution vary from state to state, but usually the prescriber, patient, and pharmacist must agree before a generic product is dispensed in place of a brand name product. If the prescription is written generically, then the generic can usually be dispensed. However, if the prescription is written for the brand name product, and marked "may substitute," the patient should be asked if he or she prefers the generic name or brand name product. Because not all drugs are available as generics, the technicians should be familiar with which generics are available. When unsure of the availability, the technician should ask if the patient prefers the generic product if one is available. In certain cases, it is important to inform the patient that some insurance plans will not cover brand name products when a generic is available or that insurance plan may require higher copay for brand name products.

After the prescription has been received, the next step is to enter it into the pharmacy computer system. The basic process of keying in the patient and prescription information and generating a label should be the same despite differing software systems across pharmacies. Additionally, most insurance plans are on-line, which allows for virtually immediate responses to the pharmacy's insurance claims.

Other Jobs for Pharmacy Technicians

While many pharmacy technicians work in pharmacies, there are several other related positions in pharmaceutical business. Some of these are listed here:

- *Pharmacy business management operators.* Pharmacy management companies are beginning to realize the importance of knowing not only the trade and generic names of drugs but also the classifications of drugs. They are hiring technicians, rather than registered pharmacists, to help pharmacy customers over the phone, which saves money for the company.

- *Computer support technicians.* Large companies that supply hospitals, community pharmacies, and other facilities with automated medication dispensing systems are employing technicians as support personnel.

- *Software writers.* Technicians may be hired to use their terminology and drug knowledge in creating new software programs.

- *Authors.* Technicians with additional education background and extensive knowledge of pharmacy can participate not only in preparing and presenting continuing education credits but also in writing textbooks for pharmacy technicians.

- *Poison control call center operators.* Some poison control centers are using technicians to triage calls coming into the 911 stations. If the call is in regard to something life-threatening, then technicians transfer the call to a pharmacist or poison specialist. If the call is something less critical, technicians are authorized to take the call.

- *Clinical coordinators.* Responsibilities include monitoring patients who are taking specific medications and those who have conditions such as asthma. Technicians in this position may schedule patients for educational classes or refer them to the pharmacist or doctor if necessary.
- *Directors or instructors.* Pharmacy technicians can oversee technician training programs or instruct in schools around the country. Some require a Bachelor of Science degree or vocational education teaching credentials.

Efficiency and Error Prevention

Pharmacy laws are designed to protect the public by ensuring that knowledgeable individuals double-check the prescribing process and oversee the use of medications, thus preventing medication errors. The law requires a licensed pharmacist to be on duty during pharmacy business hours. Licensed pharmacists must graduate from an accredited school of pharmacy, pass a licensure examination, and pass the state pharmacy examination to practice pharmacy in that state.

Another system designed to prevent medication errors is a multiple check system. This can include a pharmacist reviewing a physician order; a pharmacy technician preparing a medication for the pharmacist to check, a nurse inspecting the dose from the pharmacy, and a patient asking questions and examining the medication before taking it.

Computer technology plays an integral role in assisting in the safe and efficient administration of healthcare. Although computers can be expensive investments for businesses, they generally improve the efficiency, productivity, and accuracy of work in the pharmacy and reduce the overall costs associated with common pharmacy tasks. To capitalize on the investment and avoid loss of information and damage to equipment due to improper use, many institutions designate a knowledgeable person to mange the computer system and serve as a resource to staff.

Bar codes can help healthcare teams to ensure that the patients receive the correct drug and dosage via the correct route and at the correct time. Bar codes are unique arrangements of lines used to identify the items on which they are printed. Bart coding medications identifies the drug name, strength, dosage form, lot number, and expiration date of a particular drug product. To translate the bar code, a hand-held or fixed-position scanner is needed. Some community and institutional pharmacies use bar codes to save time and promote accuracy when performing tasks such as ordering, distributing, returning inventory, billing patients for drug dispensed, crediting patients for returned drugs, and filling and checking unit-dose carts.

The pharmacy must weigh all the costs associated with implementing new technology against the expected benefit in terms of improved quality, safety and efficiency, before deciding to put new equipment into practice. These technologies require informed, educated operators who understand how the technology can be used. The goal should be to increase quality and reduce errors in the most cost-effective manner. Automation can allow departments to maintain or increase the level of service without significant changes in staffing. The use of technology is much more likely to change the scope of technician's responsibilities than result in job elimination. Current computer technology used in healthcare includes:

- bar coding
- touch screens
- light pens
- voice recognition
- medication packagers and unit-dose appointment systems
- automated dispensing systems

- process control devices
- paperless charting

Pharmacy departments are responsible for managing their resources effectively and controlling costs. Computers allow management and staff to generate reports that can help evaluate and improve workflow and medication use. These reports give the management the opportunity to analyze and interpret data more thoroughly. Some common and valuable reports used by management include

- monitoring non formulary drug use
- drug use patterns
- drug costs
- productivity
- workload
- pharmacist intervention

Intervention data can be useful for justifying clinical pharmacist positions or additional resources. The most useful report details the type of intervention, time spent, dollar impact, and significance of the intervention. Unfortunately, most systems do not have built-in reports, so they must be written or developed by the pharmacy department.

Customer Satisfaction

All pharmaceutical businesses have customers. As you strive to increase customer satisfaction at your place of employment, consider the following tips to help improve pharmacy service:

- *Know your customer.* Being able to identify different customer types is an important first step in anticipating customer needs and managing the expectations of each person.
- *Practice good communication.* Regardless of customer type, nothing works better in terms of managing customer expectations than basic communication.
- *Know your scope of practice.* Some tasks may be performed only by the pharmacist, other are the responsibility of the pharmacy technician. Efficient workflow and good customer service rely on everyone in the pharmacy understanding his or her role.

Chapter Summary

- Pharmaceutical businesses are responsible for researching, production, and marketing of pharmaceutical supplies all over the world. They are responsible for giving the proper and safe drug therapy for different patients with specific medical needs.
- The pharmaceutical market and sciences are growing, meaning pharmaceutical businesses and pharmacies must operate efficiently and making use of available technology.
- Legal, ethical, and professional requirements must be observed in all pharmaceutical businesses and pharmacies. Policies and procedures must be made readily available to relevant staff.
- There are several pharmacy settings, including community pharmacies, managed care pharmacies, and mail-order pharmacies.
- Technology plays an important role in assuring safe and efficient administration of healthcare by increasing the quality of the products and reducing errors in a

cost-effective manner. Computers allow management and staff to generate reports that can help evaluate and improve workflow and medication use.

• Pharmacy personnel can take an active role in ensuring customer satisfaction by understanding the customer, communicating well, and knowing their scope of practice.

PRACTICE TEST QUESTIONS

Business Management

1. There are four main associations concerned with pharmacy practice. Which one listed is *not* a member?
   a. ASHP
   b. APhA
   c. JACHO
   d. AAPT

2. What job responsibility for a technician is found in an inpatient setting, but not in a community setting?
   a. insurance billing technician
   b. IV technician
   c. stock inventory technician
   d. technician recruiter

3. Healthcare institutions are usually organized into several levels of management. Which position is not at the top of the institution?
   a. department managers
   b. CEO
   c. COO
   d. CFO

4. Policy and procedures manuals exist for which of the following reason(s)?
   a. to serve as a legal document
   b. to prevent error caused by verbal communication
   c. to train new employees
   d. all of the above

5. The definition of a *policy* is:
   a. a way of accomplishing something or acting
   b. a definite course or method of action selected from among alternatives; a high-level, overall plan
   c. a series of steps followed in a regular definite order
   d. a traditional or established way of doing things.

6. The Clinical Section of the policy and procedure manual contains those activities involved in patient-related monitoring activities of a clinical nature. Which activity listed is *not* part of this section?
   a. drug ordering
   b. unit-dose drug distribution
   c. drug information services
   d. formulary operation

7. A not-for-profit, nongovernmental corporation whose responsibility is to regulate hospital settings is:
   a. JCAHO
   b. OSHA
   c. ASHP
   d. NABP

8. The definition of *procedure* is:
   a. a high-level, overall plan embracing the general goals
   b. a traditional or established way of doing things
   c. a definite course or method of action
   d. none of the above

9. Regulations affecting pharmacy practice encompass:
   a. CSA regulations
   b. JCAHO standards
   c. federal and state rules
   d. all of the above

10. The Administrative section of a policy and procedure manual contain all the following information *except*:
    a. department's hours of operation
    b. inventory control
    c. drug therapy monitoring
    d. annual reports

11. Policy and procedure manuals have a standard format. The first item in the manual is:
    a. title
    b. table of contents
    c. objectives
    d. goals

12. The liaison between the medical staff and the department of pharmacy services is:
    a. JCAHO
    b. The pharmacy and Therapeutics Committee
    c. Medicare
    d. hospital Board of Pharmacy

13. Pharmacy technicians perform essential tasks that do not require:
    a. computer entry training
    b. compounding techniques

c. label preparation

d. the pharmacist's skill or expertise

14. Pharmacy technicians may use the following designation after their name after passing the Pharmacy Technician National Certification exam:

a. APhT

b. CPhT

c. RTech

d. CPT

15. The members of the Pharmacy & Therapeutic committee review and update the manual every:

a. year

b. two years

c. 5 years

d. 18 months

16. The State Boards of Pharmacy have the responsibility of:

a. dealing with complaints

b. licensure and registration of pharmacy staff

c. poison schedules

d. all of the above

17. Which of the following is *not* true regarding policy and procedure manuals?

a. any change in the manual requires the approval of the CEO

b. they provide job descriptions for new employees

c. they guarantee accuracy in routine operational activities

d. they prevent waste of time by providing direction in repetitive tasks

18. The OBRA '90 requires community pharmacists offer:

a. free samples if the patient cannot afford the medication

b. counseling to Medicaid patients regarding their medication

c. ordering of all medications

d. inventory control

19. One of the most positive responses to a dissatisfied a customer is:

a. listening intently

b. making eye contact

c. restating what the customer has to say

d. all of the above

20. If the technician is unable to resolve the customer's problem, he/she should:

a. inform the pharmacist

b. ask another technician for help

c. ask to speak to another family member of the customer

d. ask the customer to leave

14

Professionalism and Personnel Management

Test Topics

After completing this chapter, you should be able to demonstrate knowledge of the following:

1. Communication within an organization
2. Principles of resource allocation
3. Required operational licenses and certificates
4. Roles and responsibilities of pharmacists, pharmacy technicians, and other pharmacy employees
5. Legal and regulatory requirements for personnel, facilities, equipment, and supplies
6. Professional standards for personnel, facilities, equipment, and supplies
7. Quality improvement standards and guidelines
8. State board of pharmacy regulations
9. Staff training techniques
10. Employee performance evaluation and feedback techniques

Test Terms

- **legend** a drug that can be dispensed to the public only with an order given by a properly authorized person
- **medical orders** the means of communication between the pharmacy and physicians in an institutional setting whereby medical procedures and prescription medications are described
- **pharmacy satellite** a designated area with patient care where drugs are stored, prepared, and dispensed for patients
- **policies and procedures (P&P)** documents provided by an institution to give guidance to personnel regarding what is expected of them
- **quality control** the process of checks and balances followed during the manufacturing of a product or the delivery of a service to ensure that the end product or services meets or exceeds previously determined standards
- **quality improvement** a scientific and systematic process involving monitoring, evaluating, and identifying problems and then developing and measuring the improvement strategies
- **registration** the process of being enrolled in an existing list of accepted pharmacy technicians who have met the standards of a particular state

Managing the oversight and administration of hospital and community pharmacies requires policies, procedures, regulations, and training. Federal, state, local, and institution-based laws and guidelines work together to make the practice of pharmacy safe, quality-controlled, and accountable. Before you ever pick up a counting plate or hold a patient's medical order in your hands, steps will have been taken to educate, train, and advise you of the expectations that you must meet in order to maintain your responsibilities.

There are federal and state agencies that oversee and mandate laws that govern pharmacy practice, and within an institution, there are policies and procedures as well. How will you know how to use the computer system? Do you have to pass a national pharmacy technician examination? Who evaluates your performance, and how frequently? What recourse do you have if you've been under-trained, mismanaged, or ill-advised? There are checks and balances in place to help you be a successful pharmacy technician, but some of the initial effort can only come from you. Just like anything worth doing, being aware of your responsibilities and being proactive in the management of your career are key components in becoming a confident, reliable pharmacy technician.

Professional Oversight

Before working in a pharmacy environment, you must be somewhat knowledgeable of the laws that govern the practice of pharmacy. As you learned in Chapter 2, there are federal, state, and local laws, as well as institutional guidelines, that shape pharmacy practice. Federal laws govern all 50 states, but individual states pass laws specific to the practice within their borders, and these laws may differ from one another. When you're unsure of what law prevails, the most stringent or strictest law is the one to be followed.

Standards

There are standards that direct the training, licensing, and certification of pharmacies and those who work within them. These standards are mandated by federal, state, and local laws, as well as by the institutions that employ such personnel.

Pharmacy Technicians

Although training requirements vary from state to state and from employer to employer, most pharmacy technicians are required to have obtained at least a high-school diploma. Again, between states and organizations, the level of training a technician must have varies. However, several professional groups, including the American Society of Health-System Pharmacists (ASHP), the American Pharmaceutical Association (APhA), the American Association of Colleges of Pharmacy (AACP), and the National Association of Boards of Pharmacy (NABP), came together to analyze what pharmacy technicians do and what knowledge they needed to perform their tasks. In 1995, the Pharmacy Technician Certification Board (PTCB) was founded, and it developed a voluntary national pharmacy technician certification program. They created four goals for pharmacy technicians:

• To work more effectively with the pharmacist
• To provide greater patient care and service
• To create a minimum standard of knowledge
• To help employers determine knowledge base

An increasing number of states are acknowledging the need for standards and training to ensure that the technicians who are hired are competent in all areas of pharmacy, so vocational schools, community colleges, and technical schools are offering programs to prepare students for the national exam. To take the exam in most states, an applicant need only have a high-school diploma (or general equivalency diploma) and never been convicted of a drug-related felony.

More and more states are requiring the **registration** of pharmacy technicians. Registration is the process of being enrolled in an existing list of accepted pharmacy technicians who have met the standards of a particular state. Registration is an important rule for pharmacy management that ensures that each technician has a clean background to work in a pharmacy environment.

Despite differences in registration and certification requirements between states, there are some job expectations that are universal, including the following:

• Handling incoming pharmacy telephone calls from patients, providers, and physicians under a pharmacist's supervision

- Troubleshooting third-party prescription claims
- Entering orders and patient information into a computer system
- Providing drug information to patients, nurses, and physicians
- Verifying the completeness of a physician's medical order or prescription
- Filling and initialing prescriptions

In all situations, technicians may only work under the supervision of a pharmacist, and the pharmacist is ultimately responsible for the technician's performance and activities. Were something to be prepared incorrectly, the pharmacist is liable and therefore must approve the pharmacy technician's work. Only pharmacists may counsel patients on medications, so always defer to the pharmacist when a patient inquires about their medication or about an over-the-counter drug.

Pharmacists

Pharmacists earn either a B.S. in Pharmacy or a Pharm.D. degree and then are required to pass their state's board of pharmacy examination. Once they pass their state board exam, they become a registered pharmacist (R.Ph.) and are allowed to practice pharmacy in their state. Each state has its own board that registers and regulates the practice of pharmacy, so pharmacists may be required to take a state board examination again if they move to another state.

State Pharmacy Boards

Each state has its own pharmacy board, which is composed of pharmacists and members of the public who have been appointed to the board by the state's governor. Their job is to protect the state's citizens by

- passing pharmacy rules and regulations,
- overseeing the rules passed by the state's legislature, and
- licensing pharmacists who practice in their state.

Some state pharmacy boards institute regulations for pharmacy technicians as well. These regulations can be found on the state board's website. The boards are the bodies that may require pharmacy technician registration.

Legal and Regulatory Requirements

As you learned in Chapter 2, the FDA and DEA oversee and enact the enforcement of federal laws pertaining to the practice of pharmacy. Most federal laws apply mainly to retail pharmacy, but variations of these laws apply to hospital and long-term care settings as well.

Records and Labeling

Hospital, home health, and community pharmacies differ in the type and length of time that patient records should be kept. However, all must keep complete and accurate records of their patients. All of these must maintain the following information:

- Patient's full name
- Prescriber's name
- Name and strength of drug
- Date of issue
- Expiration date
- Directions on how to take the drug (i.e. once daily)

Community and home health pharmacies also must maintain

- Prescription number
- Lot and control number of drug
- Drug manufacturer

The state pharmacy boards require that all medication that leaves the pharmacy must be checked by a pharmacist, initialed by a technician, and packaged in a proper container. Packaging issues are particularly important, and there are guidelines for these as well.

Packaging

The 1970 Poison Prevention Packaging Act requires manufacturers and pharmacies to dispense drugs in containers with childproof caps, including both over-the-counter and **legend** drugs. There are exceptions to this law, however. A non-childproof cap may be used if:

- the patient's physician requests it
- the medication requires a non-childproof cap
- the medication is for a hospitalized patient
- the patient specifically requests it

Some of the drugs that do not require childproof packaging include:

- nitroglycerin
- oral contraceptives
- prednisone
- betamethasone
- sodium fluoride

Facilities Management

Retail (community) pharmacies typically operate as free-standing entities, selling drugs and filling prescriptions directly for the public. These can be found as pharmacy-only stores or those that are part of a grocery or warehouse-type store. Although pharmacists counsel patients in this setting, the institutional setting (hospital, nursing home, long-term care facility) is the more intricate, patient-centered setting where patients receive their care in a structured manner. The organization and management of these types of facilities are crucial to providing optimal patient care, and the institutional pharmacy plays a big part in the system.

Resources

In an institutional pharmacy setting, the pharmacy is a significant entity in the flow of patient care. Healthcare institutions, such as hospitals, are organized into several levels of management. The manner in which the pharmacy is utilized in these settings varies, but the goal is always quality patient care.

Technology

As you learned in Chapter 12, technology, including the use of computers and robotic systems, increases the efficiency, quality, and accountability in the pharmacy. Pharmacy technicians master the use of computer systems to input patient profile information; interpret and fill **medical orders**, the most common method of communication between the pharmacy and physicians; and communicate with other departments. The use of unit-dose machines and their upkeep is often the job of the pharmacy technician. Depending on the type of pharmacy services that the institution provides, pharmacy technicians will perform specific tasks.

Centralized Pharmacy Services

From a central location, centralized pharmacy services handle:

- pharmacy personnel
- resources
- functions of the pharmacy

They're often located in hospital basements, and from there, they:

- prepare IV medications
- stock medication carts
- attend to medical orders
- service an outpatient prescription counter
- store and stock medications and supplies

Centralized pharmacy services have some disadvantages, however, including the lack of face-to-face interactions with patients and other healthcare providers and the time it takes to deliver medication to the far reaches of the institution. Even patient records are difficult to access for the pharmacists, who are tasked with making appropriate therapeutic assessments of medication orders for patients.

A pharmacy technician in a centralized pharmacy can expect to perform tasks such as:

- preparing IVs, hyperalimentation, and chemotherapeutic agents
- filling patient medication carts
- delivering narcotics
- restocking drugs for medication dispensing systems
- compounding products not available from a manufacturer
- functions related to quality control and improvement
- billing
- completing miscellaneous paperwork

Decentralized Pharmacy Services

Decentralized pharmacies work in tandem with centralized pharmacies. These services are provided from within a patient care area, such as a **pharmacy satellite**, which is a designated area with patient care where drugs are stored, prepared, and dispensed for patients. These satellites are typically staffed by one or more pharmacists and pharmacy technicians. Their proximity to patients and other healthcare providers allows the pharmacist to interact directly with patients, thereby:

- obtaining pertinent information.
- monitoring and assessing a patient's drug therapy response.
- disseminating patient education materials.
- answering drug information questions.

The greatest disadvantage to a decentralized pharmacy is its level of resource requirement. Because it's operating separately and in addition to a centralized pharmacy, it must be staffed with additional pharmacists and pharmacy technicians; stocked with medications, supplies, and references; and outfitted with such equipment as a laminar flow hood, computers, and printers.

In a satellite setting, the pharmacy technician's jobs may include:

- maintaining medication and supply inventory
- rotating expired medication out of stock
- cleaning and maintaining laminar flow hoods
- preparing unit-dose and IV medication orders in a timely fashion
- occasionally answering questions from nurses and making judgments on when to refer a question to the pharmacist

RECALL TIP

To help you remember the difference between centralized and decentralized pharmacy services, remember that centralized are centered in an institution layout, while decentralized services are dispersed throughout the patient care units.

Quality Standards

As you learned in Chapter 12, quality control and improvement is a key factor in providing a high level of patient care. Without the proper procedures and guidelines in place to ensure quality, contamination, adverse effects, and even death can occur. The costs of ensuring quality are outweighed by the benefit to the patient and to the healthcare system as a whole, because errors in quality control can lead to significant financial consequences for both individuals and institutions. The Joint Commission on Accreditation of Healthcare Organizations (JCAHO) have made quality a high-priority issue for institutional practices.

Quality Control

Quality control is the process of checks and balances followed during the manufacturing of a product or the delivery of a service to ensure that the end product or services meets or exceeds previously determined standards, with the goal of zero errors and zero problems. A quality control program includes:

- written policies and procedures
- training for staff who participate in the procedure
- checks and balances at critical points of the process

Quality control is particularly important in the preparation of intravenous medications, as an error in drug concentration or in the process of preparation that introduces contamination may cause illness or death in a patient.

A disadvantage to quality control programs is the significant cost in both time and resources that is added to the process. It does identify errors and defects, but it doesn't always uncover the underlying cause of a problem.

RECALL TIP

What's your greatest ally in the accomplishment of quality control? Other pharmacy technicians. Rechecking one another's work, especially in IV preparation, will improve your quality and confidence in these types of preparations. Remember that a quick check = quality control.

Quality Improvement

Quality improvement is a scientific and systematic process involving monitoring, evaluating, and identifying problems and then developing and measuring the improvement strategies. Quality improvement focuses on problems, not people, and it requires that decisions are based on factual data. Tools are required to identify the problems, assist in the data collection, and then analyze the findings or data. Useful tools in a quality improvement program include:

- *Brainstorming* — ideas, problems, and solutions
- *Workflow diagram* — showing the steps of a particular procedure
- *Run chart* — a statistical tool that tracks patterns and trends over a period of time

Accrediting agencies such as the JCAHO require pharmacies to participate in quality improvement programs. You as a pharmacy technician are invaluable in a successful quality improvement program by:

- preparing surveys or inspections for the JCAHO
- ensuring refrigeration logs are completed
- inspecting medication units
- inspecting IV hoods regularly
- maintaining databases for adverse drug reaction reports, medication occurrence reports, and drug use evaluations

Personnel Training and Evaluations

A key element in any service industry is the people who provide the service and their level of training, competency, and expertise. Technology is a wonderfully useful addition to pharmacy practice, but it is no replacement for the human touch, especially as it pertains to interactions with patients and providers.

Communication

RECALL TIP

To inspire confidence in your position, it's a good idea to "dress up"—not in your Sunday's best, but dress as though you held the next level position in your pharmacy. You'll improve your confidence while inviting patients, pharmacists, and physicians to take you seriously.

Pharmacy technicians are often the first-line communicators in a pharmacy. You answer the phone, you consult with the pharmacist, you attend to patient requests, and you receive prescriptions, medical orders, and other written instructions. The way others perceive you has an impact on the confidence they have in you. That's what it's very important that in your written, oral, and physical communication (e.g., body language), you present yourself as a professional with confidence, compassion, and patience. People make an instant judgment of you based on your body language.

Leaving your personal problems behind you when you cross the threshold of the pharmacy will go a long way in ensuring everyone that your top priority is the business at hand. Be conscious of your facial expressions and posture, and make an effort to appear helpful and concerned for the situation at hand. Learning to communicate effectively without ever using words is an invaluable skill that is worthwhile to master.

Training

All pharmacy personnel, including pharmacists and pharmacy technicians, require training. Knowing the inner workings of a particular pharmacy setting will ensure the smooth accomplishment of your daily tasks. Training occurs both initially, upon hiring, and as continuing education when new systems or procedures are brought into practice.

Policies and Procedures

All pharmacies operate under the direction of documentation known as **policies and procedures** (P&P). These documents give guidance for the personnel regarding what is expected of them. P&P are typically contained in reference manual that is readily available to all personnel. The JCAHO requires that pharmacy departments develop P&P manuals. General P&P manuals set forth for a particular institution or retail pharmacy company contain information such as:

- Hiring requirements
- Employee benefits
- Employee orientation, training, and evaluation

A pharmacy-specific P&P manual will provide information that directly relates to the operations of the pharmacy department. Such a manual provides information concerning the delivery of efficient, quality drug therapy and may include sections covering:

- the correct aseptic technique for compounding medications or IV admixtures
- monitoring patients with drug allergies
- handling procedures for chemotherapeutic agents
- distribution and control of all drugs
- use of investigational drugs
- management of toxic or dangerous drugs
- provision for pharmacy services in the event of a disaster
- management of pharmacy expenditures and the pharmacy's budget

Pharmacy P&P manuals are developed by the pharmacy director who receives input from pharmacists, physicians, or other healthcare professionals. They're reviewed by a committee before implementation, and they're typically reviewed and updated annually. The P&P manuals are the primary source for all procedural details in a pharmacy or institution; no memo, e-mail, or second-hand communication can take its place.

RECALL TIP

P&P manuals provide you with all the tools you need to answer questions about your job and the company for whom you work. P&P can also stand for partnering and progressing – two descriptive words describing your career if you follow the P&Ps.

Roles and Responsibilities

Upon applying for a pharmacy technician position, you will be interviewed by not only the pharmacy department manager but also a representative from the institution's or company's human resources department. This employee will be able to give you a broad overview of how the organization runs and the workflow within it. This is an opportunity for you to ask questions about growth, benefits, evaluations, holiday and salary information, and any other non–pharmacy-related questions. Once you've been hired, you will probably receive training from a pharmacy technician supervisor. This person usually has a great deal of experience both in the field and in the company or institution and will aid you in your transition into the department.

Most of the positions held by pharmacy technicians are in retail settings, but some are in institutional or hospital pharmacies. In the pharmacy P&P manual for your organization, you will find descriptions of all positions in the department, from pharmacy director to pharmacy technician, and all of the functions and tasks required for each position. Even within the category there may be various levels of experience and training required. For example, a first-level pharmacy technician may be responsible for:

- entering medication orders in the computer system
- filling medication orders or prescriptions
- stocking medication storage shelves
- maintaining automated unit-dose systems

A second-level pharmacy technician, in addition to first-level duties, may be responsible for:

- compounding IV admixtures
- following aseptic techniques
- having mathematical ease in pharmaceutical calculations

It's important to know what position you are filling and what the responsibilities and duties entail. Often, technicians are expected to float between levels and fill in where needed, so if you are not comfortable or adept in a particular area, it would behoove you to make your supervisor aware.

Performance Evaluations

Pharmacy technicians are evaluated annually, either from their date of hire or according to the evaluation timeline of their employer. These evaluations are conducted in accordance with the contents of the pharmacy P&P manual, so there shouldn't be surprises regarding your job expectations. Evaluations are important to ensure that you are competent in all aspects of your job and that you meet or exceed the expectations that your supervisor has of you. A great place to find the expectations for your job is in the pharmacy's P&P manual, which details the functions and tasks of your position, the authority of the position (who reports to whom), and dress code or appearance expectations for your position. Performance evaluations often result in salary increases and occasionally in promotion or added responsibilities. The more opportunities you have to try different aspects of the pharmacy technician job, the better-rounded an employee you are, and therefore are more valuable to the organization.

What if you have questions, concerns, or a disagreement with the evaluation you receive? The best time to discuss this is at the end of your evaluation. Supervisors should function as both mentors and guides in the business for you, and they're not your enemy. They want to see you succeed, since that will make their job less stressful as well as contribute to the overall success of the pharmacy. If you think you need additional training, would like to try a new duty, or if you are uncomfortable with an aspect of your job, the evaluation time is the time to bring it forward. If you aren't forthright, you'll become frustrated with your job. Use your supervisor as a resource, mentor, and ally, and you'll be able to work out any problems that you encounter.

RECALL TIP
Remember the ABCs of your yearly evaluation: Ask questions, Be attentive, and seek Criticism. You'll be perceived as respectful, having initiative, and seeking feedback that will improve your standing as an employee.

Chapter Summary

- Federal, state, and local laws govern the practice of pharmacy.
- When laws conflict, the most stringent law prevails.
- The PTCB developed national standards for pharmacy technicians, who can be certified by passing an examination.
- Some states require pharmacy technicians to register with their board of pharmacy in order to be employed in their state.
- Pharmacists register through a state's board of pharmacy after passing the state's board examination to receive their license to practice pharmacy.
- State pharmacy boards oversee the pharmacy rules and regulations and license pharmacists.
- Each institution has requirements for labeling, packaging, and storage of patient and drug information in accordance with state and federal law.
- Medical orders are the means of communication between the pharmacy and physicians in an institutional setting whereby medical procedures and prescription medications are described.
- Centralized pharmacy services prepare medical orders and fill prescriptions from a hospital's basement.
- Decentralized pharmacy services work in tandem with centralized pharmacy services to provide care from a patient area known as a satellite pharmacy.
- Quality control is necessary to ensure that previously determined standards are met or exceeded.

- Quality improvement seeks to solve root problems that may affect quality in an institution and is often assessed by the JCAHO.
- Effective physical, written, and oral communication with patients, pharmacists, nurses, and physicians is the key to success in the pharmacy.
- On-the-job training occurs initially and as needs arise for continuing education.
- Policies and procedures dictate the operations of the organization and the expectations of the personnel.
- Pharmacy technicians are evaluated annually based on the expectations laid out in the pharmacy's P&P manual for competency and job satisfaction.

PRACTICE TEST QUESTIONS

Professionalism and Personnel Management

1. Which of the following statements about quality control is *false*?
   a. Quality control is necessary for IV products because of morbidity and mortality.
   b. Written policies and procedures are not necessary if a quality control format is in place.
   c. Quality control builds checks and balances.
   d. All of the above

2. Which of the following statements regarding quality improvement is *false*?
   a. It is an important part of preparation for a JCAHO survey.
   b. It concentrates on problems within the system.
   c. The pharmacy director is totally responsible for quality improvement.
   d. All of the above

3. Laws governing pharmacists, technicians, and other pharmacy personnel are set by
   a. individual state laws
   b. the NABP
   c. the pharmacy itself
   d. professional organizations

4. The organization that certifies pharmacy technicians is
   a. ASHP
   b. NABP
   c. PTCB
   d. APhA

5. Memos can be substituted for policy and procedure updates.
   a. True
   b. False

6. Technicians should familiarize themselves with the administrative and technical aspects of the policy and procedure manual.

   a. True
   b. False

7. The primary goal of pharmacy personnel is communication not only with customers but also with other professionals. Which form of communication is judged by others in the first 30 seconds of meeting?
   a. listening skills
   b. appearance
   c. phone skills
   d. body language

8. Most pharmacies that hire technicians require the same basic skills. Which skill listed is *not* the responsibility of a technician?
   a. troubleshooting third-party prescription claim questions
   b. handling ongoing pharmacy telephone calls
   c. counseling patients on OTC medications
   d. taking in refill prescriptions

9. Many states have laws that differ from federal laws. Pharmacy personnel need to remember
   a. always follow the state law
   b. always follow the strictest law
   c. always follow the federal law
   d. depends on the situation

10. Technicians are monitored in their job performance competency through regularly scheduled performance reviews.
    a. True
    b. False

11. Which system allows for a closer relationship between the pharmacist and medical team, including the patient?
    a. centralized system
    b. decentralized system

c. floor stock system
d. individual prescription orders

12. Although statutes, regulations and standards of practice vary from state to state, under all circumstances, the technician is expected to
    a. work under the supervision of the pharmacist
    b. follow FDA guidelines regarding drug storage
    c. counsel patients on OTC medications
    d. review patient profiles for interactions

13. Technicians have several methods for performance feedback after an evaluation. The most effective method is
    a. faxing your concerns to your supervisor
    b. by preparing a memo
    c. airing your concerns at the time of the evaluation
    d. leaving your concerns on a voice message

14. The most common routine method of communication in the hospital between the pharmacy and the physician is a
    a. prescription
    b. medical order
    c. fax
    d. telephone

15. The State Board of Pharmacy requires that all medication leaving the pharmacy must
    a. be packaged in a proper container
    b. be checked by a pharmacist

c. be initialed by a technician
d. all of the above

16. All pharmacy employees are required to be interviewed not only by the pharmacy department by also with
    a. human resources
    b. security
    c. administration
    d. housekeeping

17. Technician training in the pharmacy is usually performed by
    a. the pharmacy manager
    b. outside training coordinator
    c. technician supervisor
    d. none of the above

18. The Policy and Procedure Manual contains information pertaining to
    a. disciplinary actions
    b. performance evaluations
    c. step-by-step directions on how to perform various tasks
    d. all of the above

19. Performance evaluations are usually conducted
    a. monthly
    b. yearly on the technician's starting date
    c. twice a year
    d. bimonthly

15

Infection Control and Hazardous Materials

Test Topics

After completing this chapter, you should be able to demonstrate knowledge of the following:

1. Infection control procedures
2. Requirements for handling hazardous products and disposing of hazardous waste
3. Documentation requirements for controlled substances, investigational drugs, and hazardous wastes
4. Storage and handling requirements for hazardous substances (for example, chemotherapeutics, radiopharmaceuticals)
5. Hazardous waste disposal requirements
6. Procedures for the treatment of exposure to hazardous substances (for example, eyewash)
7. Laminar flow hood maintenance requirements
8. Infection control policies and procedures
9. Sanitation requirements (for example: hand washing, cleaning, counting trays, countertop, and equipment)

Test Terms

- **body substance isolation** the practice of isolating all body substances (blood, urine, feces, tears, etc.) of individuals who might be infected with illnesses to reduce the chances of transmitting these illnesses
- **disinfection** the use of liquid chemicals on surfaces and at room temperature to kill disease-causing microorganisms
- **explosive substances** release sudden pressure, gaseous elements, and heat when subjected to shock, hot or high pressure
- **flammable and combustible substances** those that are easy to ignite, for example paint thinners, charcoal, lighter fluid, and silver polish
- **hazardous material** any substance or mixture of substances having properties capable of producing adverse effects on the health and safety or the environment of a human being
- **infection control** factors related to the spread of infections within the healthcare setting
- **infectious waste** includes blood, blood products and body fluids, infectious sharps waste, laboratory waste, and animal waste
- **investigational product** a pharmaceutical form of an active ingredient or placebo tested and used as a reference in a clinical trial
- **personal protective equipment (PPE)** specialized clothing or equipment worn by healthcare workers for protection against a hazard by creating a physical barrier
- **poisons** also known as or toxic materials, can cause injury or death when they enter the bodies of living things
- **radiopharmaceuticals** unique medicinal formulations containing radioisotopes used in major clinical areas for diagnosis and/or therapy
- **standard precautions** are the minimum required level of infection control in all settings and all situations, and thus define safe work practices regardless of known or presumed infectious status

- **sterilization** a process intended to kill all microorganisms and is the highest level of microbial kill that is possible
- **solid waste** a term used by the U.S. Environmental Protection Agency (EPA) to define all solid, liquid, and gaseous waste

The Federal Food, Drug, and Cosmetic Act of 1938 recognized United States Pharmacopeia (USP) 797 as the official compendium of drug standards. Today, USP is the official public standards-setting authority for all prescription and over-the-counter medicines, dietary supplements, and other healthcare products manufactured and sold in the United States.

The intent of USP is to prevent harm to patients that could result from microbial and endotoxin contamination, large content errors in the strength of correct ingredients, and incorrect ingredients. Patients receiving compounded sterile doses of chemotherapy and other injectable hazardous drugs are at high risk for errors addressed by USP. Chemotherapy drugs are very potent, and small errors in calculation or reconstitution during compounding can lead to serious harm.

Daily preparation and compounding of various medications requires knowledge of aseptic technique (see Chapter 9). Although pharmacists are responsible for all medications dispensed from the pharmacy, they cannot watch every pharmacy technician every moment of the day to ensure that proper procedures are used. Competent pharmacy technicians have learned how to use aseptic technique and why it is important to cultivate their skills. Pharmacy supervisors periodically take samples of compounded intravenous drugs and send them to the laboratory to test for microbial growth. Because each sample is accompanied by the name of the pharmacy technician who prepared it, this information maybe used to assess his or her performance.

Infection Control Procedures

Germs in our bodies cause infection. **Infection control** addresses factors related to the spread of infections within the healthcare setting, including education and prevention, proper monitoring, management, and the investigation of demonstrated or suspected spread of infection within a particular healthcare setting.

Infections in a healthcare setting can easily spread from person to person. There are three types of infection transmission possible:

1. Airborne transmission (for example, pulmonary tuberculosis)
2. Droplet transmission (for example, influenza)
3. Contact transmission (for example, skin ulcers)

As a pharmacy technician, you will be trained on proper infection control for the facility in which you work.

Handling and Disposing of Hazardous Products and Waste

Solid waste is a term used by the U.S. Environmental Protection Agency (EPA) to define all solid, liquid, and gaseous waste. Hazardous and infectious chemicals and medical wastes are subcategories of solid waste that can threaten human health or the environment because they may be potentially harmful.

Hazardous material is any substance or mixture of substances having properties capable of producing adverse effects on the health and safety or the environment of a human being. Hazardous materials include substances, chemical and medical wastes.

Medical waste is sometimes referred to as "red-bag waste" or "infectious waste." **Infectious waste** includes blood, blood products and body fluids, infectious sharps waste, laboratory waste, and animal waste (contaminated and noncontaminated).

Controlled Substances

The task of counting, dispensing, and tracking controlled substances is a critical job that requires perfection. In each hospital unit that stocks controlled substances, two nurses must conduct an actual count at the change of every shift. Therefore, all controlled substances are accounted for three times daily. Controlled substances in most cases are kept in a locked cabinet such as a Pyxis, MedDispense or some type of computerized dispensing machine. Authorized personnel are assigned a user identification security code such as a password or fingerprint that is scanned and verified before the system grants access.

Some essential drugs used in medical practices are considered acutely hazardous waste or "P-listed" waste, and thus, require proper labeling and regulation. The facility must dispose of unused preparations of these as hazardous waste or as "universal waste."

DEA Order Forms for Schedule II Medications

For Schedule II medications, the physician writes a Schedule II prescription with all of the information required. The compounding pharmacy then prepares the medication and transfers possession to the physician. The physician must submit a DEA Form 222 Official Order Form to the compounding pharmacy along with the prescription. DEA Order Forms may be obtained online at the DEA website (www.deadiversion.usdoj.gov).

The forms must be completed in pen, in indelible pencil, or typed. The DEA 222 form is a three-part form. The pharmacy or physician's office retains the bottom copy. The top and middle copies are sent to the supplier or manufacturer. The supplier then forwards the middle copy to the DEA.

Prescriptions and Transfer Records for Controlled Substance Schedules III, IV, and V

The physician writes a Schedule III—V prescription with all of the information required. The compounding pharmacy prepares the medication and transfers possession to the physician. A transfer record is maintained at the pharmacy and the physician's office. The record must document the drug name, strength, dosage form, and quantity. A transfer form is available at the BNDD website (www.dhss.mo.gov/BNDD).

Controlled Substance Record-Keeping Requirements for Physicians

All controlled substance administrations need proper documentation in the patient's chart. When Schedule II medications are undertaken, the third copy of the DEA Order Form needs to specify the quantity of the drug received and the date of receipt. DEA Order Forms must have a separate file from all other records and must be in chronological order.

Physicians must maintain records of all controlled substances received in the practice. DEA Order Forms will document the Schedule II medications. For medications in Schedules III, IV, and V, there must be a document specifying the drug name, strength, dosage form, quantity of the drugs received, the date, and the names, addresses, and DEA numbers of both the supplier and the receiver.

Controlled Substance Record-Keeping Requirements for Pharmacies

> **RECALL TIP**
>
> Keeping the appropriate forms on file is necessary for all pharmacies to remain up-to-date on their records and in accordance with the law. Make it a habit of checking records for all controlled substance prescriptions that you fill.

The pharmacy must have separate registrations as a compounding pharmacy and a distributor. The pharmacy will have two separate DEA numbers. The two types of DEA Order Forms should also be in separate files. One file provided for the retail business papers and a separate file for the distribution and registration papers. DEA form 222 prescriptions and distribution records must be kept on file in the pharmacy for a minimum of two years.

Physicians' Destruction of Compounded Medications

There may be a need to destroy the compounded medications prescribed to a patient right on site. This must appear on the administration log for accountability. The destruction must document the date, drug name, strength, quantity wasted, and reason for the waste. Two persons should destroy the compounded medications and both of them must sign the log. All controlled substances must be destroyed beyond reclamation.

Investigational Product and Hazardous Waste

Investigational product is a pharmaceutical form of an active ingredient or placebo tested and used as a reference in a clinical trial. This includes a product with a marketing authorization when used or assembled (formulated or packaged) in a way different from the approved form, when used for an unapproved indication, or when used to gain further information about an approved use. Investigational products have not yet been approved by the FDA. Physicians or institutions conducting research are responsible for ordering investigational drugs. Pharmacy technicians are responsible for preparation, handling, inventory, storage, and record keeping of investigational drugs.

Hazardous Chemotherapeutic Waste

Chemotherapeutic (anti-neoplastic) medications and the materials used to prepare, administer, and control these materials are controlled and the waste materials are collected for special disposal. Staff using these materials are trained in the handling and emergency response to spills or leaks.

Chemotherapeutic wastes are placed inside a labeled container and transported by a contractor to an approved incinerator. If waste chemotherapeutic agents mix with infectious waste, the combined waste is secured in a red bag labeled "incinerate only."

Chemotherapeutic residual waste is handled as part of the Regulated Medical Waste stream, with additional labeling to assure appropriate incineration as final destruction. Larger than residual volumes of chemotherapeutic waste (liquids) are handled as chemical waste, if not recyclable.

Management of Radioactive Materials and Waste

Radioactive materials are labeled with the magenta and yellow symbols, defined by OSHA in the international use. These materials are handled and stored in accordance with the NRC regulations and license provisions. Radioactive waste is held in a "hot room" until decayed, and the labels are removed or defaced. It is then handled as the underlying hazard of the materials for disposal. The Radiation Safety Officer manages the waste and determines when it is no longer considered a radioactive hazard.

Management of Infectious Waste and Sharps

Regulated medical waste may be located throughout a facility. The waste management program of a given institution is designed to identify, separate, collect, and control potentially bio-hazardous materials, and to collect them for licensed disposal. Staff is trained to handle materials in the regulated medical wastes program with assistance from an Infection Control Practitioner. Labeled and specialized containers are used to collect and transport these wastes.

Regulated medical waste, including sharps, are picked up by housekeeping in patient care areas and transported to the handling room in dedicated carts. The waste is packaged for disposal, and held for a licensed waste contractor pickup. The contractor assists in completing the manifests, and removes the waste, returning the disposal copy of the manifest after final disposal.

Infectious, regulated, or bio-hazardous waste are placed in red bags in red plastic containers that labeled as "containing bio-hazardous waste."

Chemical Materials and Waste

Labels are affixed to chemical containers by the manufacturer prior to receipt, or are placed on containers by staff if filled or mixed within HSC Clinical Operations facilities.

Chemical wastes are labeled on the containers. In many cases, the waste is labeled by the original chemical name. In other cases, where collection cans or containers are used, containers are labeled as such. If the identity of the waste material is lost or uncertain, the materials are tested and analyzed to identify them for proper handling and disposal.

Radiopharmaceuticals

Radiopharmaceuticals are unique medicinal formulations containing radioisotopes used in major clinical areas for diagnosis and/or therapy. The facilities and procedures for the production, use, and storage of radiopharmaceuticals are subject to licensing by national and/or regional authorities. Regulations concerning pharmaceutical preparations include the application of current Good Manufacturing Practices (GMP).

Radiopharmaceuticals are kept in well-closed containers. The storage conditions should be such that the maximum radiation dose rate to which persons may be exposed can be reduced to an acceptable level. Radiopharmaceutical preparations that are intended for parenteral use should be kept in a glass vial, ampoule, or syringe that is sufficiently transparent to permit the visual inspection of the contents. Glass containers may darken under the effect of radiation.

Hazardous Waste Disposal

Household Hazardous Waste (HHW) is leftover household products that contain corrosive, toxic, ignitable, or reactive ingredients. Products such as paints, cleaners, oils, batteries, and pesticides that contain potentially hazardous ingredients require special care in disposing. The options of recycling, reuse, reduction, and disposal – listed in order of EPA's preferred waste management hierarchy – are all important tools to manage safely HHW.

Federal law allows disposal of house HHW in the trash. However, many communities have collection programs for HHW to reduce the potential harm posed by these chemicals. EPA encourages participation in these HHW collection programs rather than discarding the HHW in the trash. Under federal regulations, anyone generating less than 1,000 kilograms of waste chemicals per month is considered a small generator and may dispose of waste in common garbage taken to a municipal landfill or a waste facility.

As a pharmacy technician, you may be asked to help dispose of your employer's HHW. Follow the guidelines you are provided with for disposing of:

- chemical waste
- solvents
- detergents
- acids and alkalies
- metals

In addition, you may have to deal with chemical reactions of waste products that are not compatible. As a rule, do not mix or store the following chemical classes together: acids and alkalies; bleaches; oxidizing agents; reducing agents; solvents and flammables.

Treatment of Exposure to Hazardous Substances

Release of hazardous materials may occur by spilling, leaking, emitting toxic vapors, or any other process that enables the material to escape its container, enter the environment, and create a potential hazard. Classifications of different hazards are:

- **Explosive substances** release sudden pressure, gaseous elements, and heat when subjected to shock, hot or high pressure.
- **Flammable and combustible substances** are easy to ignite. Considered highly flammable are paint thinners, charcoal, lighter fluid, and silver polisher.
- **Poisons** (or toxic materials) can cause injury or death when they enter the bodies of living things.

Exposure to a toxic substance can produce either immediate or long-term effects. A reaction to a poison can occur at the time of exposure, and might include vomiting, eye irritation, or other symptoms. Long-term effects may occur years after a single serious exposure, or as the result of chronic exposure. These effects are often more difficult to trace to their cause and can include organ damage, respiratory diseases, and other illnesses. Certain toxic substances produce their long-term effects by altering the genetic code, or DNA, which tells the body's cells to perform certain activities. Three categories of effects can result from such substances:

- A carcinogenic effect is an increase in an individual's risk of contracting cancer.
- A mutagenic effect is a permanent change in the genetic material (DNA), which may pass along to later generations.
- A teratogenic effect is an increased risk that a developing embryo will have physical defects.

When the body is exposed to a toxic substance, its internal defenses try to remove the unwanted substances. The primary internal defense is excretion of the contaminant with other wastes in the feces or urine. Prior to excretion, wastes are filtered primarily by the liver and kidneys. As a result, these two organs are both subject to damage from toxic substances.

Portions of the lungs contain cilia, which try to remove particles that then may be coughed out. Particles that are too large or cannot be removed for other reasons sometimes remain as deposits in the lower part of the lungs, where they can cause toxic effects such as fibrosis or cancer.

Other body defenses against toxic substances are breathing and sweating. When an intoxicated person has the smell of alcohol on his or her breath, the smell indicates that the body is exhaling material that has no use. Tears also remove contaminants that enter the eyes.

In healthcare settings, as well as in every day life, eye emergencies, burns, and inhalation poisoning can unfortunately occur. The following sections describe basic procedures for dealing with these emergencies.

First Aid for Eye Emergencies

Knowing what to do for an eye emergency can save valuable time and possibly prevent vision loss. Following are some instructions for basic eye injury precautions and first aid.

- *Be prepared.* Wear eye protection for all hazardous activities, at home as well as and on the job. Your employer will stock a first aid kit with a rigid eye shield and commercial eyewash, so be sure you know how to use the kit before an eye injury happens. When in doubt, see a doctor immediately.

- *Chemical burns to the eye.* In all cases of eye contact with chemicals, first immediately flush the eye with water or any other drinkable liquid. Hold the eye under a faucet or shower, or pour water into the eye using a clean container. Keep the eye open and as wide as possible while flushing. Continue flushing for at least 15 minutes.

- *Specks in the eye.* Do not rub the eye. Try to let tears wash the speck out or use eyewash. Try lifting the upper eyelid outward and down over the lower lid. If the speck does not wash out, keep the eye closed, bandage it lightly, and see a doctor.

- *Blows to the eye.* Apply a cold compress without putting pressure on the eye. Crushed ice in a plastic bag may be taped to the forehead to rest gently on the injured eye.

- *Cuts and punctures of the eye or eyelid.* Do not wash out the eye with water or any other liquid. Do not try to remove an object that is stuck in the eye. Cover the eye with a rigid shield without applying pressure (for example, the bottom half of a paper cup). Seek treatment immediately.

RECALL TIP

Eye injuries can be very serious. Remember that you want to flush the eye when there is something inside like a chemical or a speck, but do not flush if the eye is cut or punctured.

First Aid for Burn

Burns destroy skin, which controls the amount of heat our bodies retain or release, holds in fluids, and protects us from infection. While burns on fingers and hands are usually not dangerous, burns injuring even relatively small areas of skin can develop serious complications. Here are the first aid steps to treat a burn:

- Treating a burn begins with stopping the burning process. Cool the burned area with cool running water for several minutes. If an ambulance is coming, continue running water over the burned area until the ambulance arrives. Look for blistering, sloughing, or charred (blackened) skin.

- Blistering and sloughing (skin coming off) mean the top layer of skin is completely damaged and complications are likely. Charring indicates even deeper damage to all three layers of skin.

- If the damaged area is bigger than one entire arm or the whole abdomen, call 911 or take the victim to the emergency department immediately. Mild burns with reddened skin and no blisters can be treated with a topical burn ointment or spray. Cool water (not cold or warm) may also help with pain.

- Do not apply butter or oil to any burn. Over the counter pain-relievers like ibuprofen or acetaminophen used for the pain of a mild burn (typically redness only). If stronger pain relief is needed, contact a physician or go to the emergency department.

- While the burn is healing, wear loose natural clothing like silks or light cottons. Harsher fabrics will irritate the skin even more.

First Aid for Inhalation Poisoning

Inhalation of toxic fumes can be very dangerous. Here are first aid steps for inhalation poisoning:

- Seek immediate emergency help
- Get help before you attempt to rescue others
- Hold a wet cloth to cover your nose and mouth or over that of the victim
- Open all the doors and windows.
- Take deep breaths before you begin the rescue
- Avoid lighting a match
- Check the patient's breathing
- Do CPR, if necessary
- If the patient vomits, take steps to prevent choking

Laminar Flow Hood

As you learned in Chapter 9, there are two types of laminar flow hoods: vertical and horizontal. The vertical hood, also known as a biology safety cabinet, is best for working with hazardous organisms since the aerosols that are generated in the hood are filtered out before they are released into the surrounding environment. Horizontal hoods are designed such that, the air flows directly at the operator. This makes them the best protection for cultures, but not useful when working with hazardous organisms.

Both types of hoods have continuous displacement of air that passes through a HEPA (high efficiency particle) filter that removes particulates from the air. In a vertical hood, the filtered air blows down from the top of the cabinet; in a horizontal hood, the filtered air blows out at the operator in a horizontal fashion. The hoods are equipped with a short-wave UV light that can be turned on for a few minutes to sterilize the surfaces of the hood. Vertical flow hoods are used in the preparation of chemotherapy medications. They have a Plexiglas shield that protects the technician from the inside work area.

The most important part of a laminar flow hood is a high efficiency bacteria-retentive filter. Room air is taken into the unit and passed through a pre-filter to remove gross contaminants. The air is then compressed and channeled up behind and through the HEPA filter (High Efficiency Particulate Air filter) in a laminar flow fashion- the purified air flows out over the entire work surface in parallel lines at a uniform velocity. The HEPA filter removes nearly all of the bacteria from the air. Both hoods must only be cleaned with 70% isopropyl alcohol.

Standard Precautions

Standard precautions define safe work practices for the care and treatment of all clients regardless of their known or presumed infectious status. It is the minimum required level of infection control in all settings and all situations. Standard precautions include the following five procedures:

1. Hand washing
2. Use of personal protective equipment
3. Correct handling and disposal of waste
4. Appropriate cleaning of client care equipment
5. Hygienic environmental control

Hand Washing

Hand washing is the single most important procedure for preventing the spread of biological contamination. Here are some hand washing tips and procedures:

1. Wet hands thoroughly all over.
2. Use pH neutral soap.
3. Lather soap all over hands.
4. Rub hands together vigorously for 15–20 seconds. Pay particular attention to the fingertips, thumbs, wrists, finger webs and the backs of the hands.
5. Rinse under running water.
6. Pat hands dry with paper towels.

There are waterless alcohol-based hand wash solutions that are as effective as soap and water hand washing. These preparations can be used when there is no visible soiling of the hands. These waterless preparations contain an emollient and aid in reducing damage to the hands.

Personal Protective Equipment (PPE)

Personal Protective Equipment (PPE) is specialized clothing or equipment worn by a worker for protection against a hazard. PPE prevents contact with a potentially infectious material by creating a physical barrier between the potential infectious material and the healthcare worker. Many or most of these items are disposable to avoid carrying infectious materials from one patient to another patient and to avoid costly disinfection.

Respiratory Protection

Masks are worn to protect you from the environment in which you work and infection from patients, or to protect patients from you if you are infectious.

- Paper mask or surgical mask: wear in areas where droplet infection of the client is a concern or when you have a cold.
- Specialized particulate respiratory filter mask: wear to protect from active pulmonary tuberculosis patients.
- Respiration mask: wear when there are noxious fumes, harmful dusts, sprays, vapors, and mists.

Foot Protection

Appropriate footwear should be worn in appropriate situations for your own safety and to prevent the spread of infection.

- Shoe covers: wear to protect from contamination when entering an area of infection.
- Enclosed, waterproof footwear with non-slip soles: wear at all times to reduce contact with blood, bodily secretions, excretions, disinfectants, or chemicals.
- Protective footwear: wear to protect from splashes, drips, and the dropping or rolling of heavy objects.

Hand and Body Protection

Many tasks in healthcare settings require that you wear gloves. There are several types of gloves for protecting your hands and for infection control.

- Sterile gloves: wear when likely to have contact with sterile body cavity.
- Non-sterile gloves: wear to reduce contact with blood, bodily secretions, excretions, disinfectants, chemicals.
- General-purpose utility gloves: wear for cleaning and during manual decontamination of used instruments and equipment.
- Heavy duty gloves: wear to reduce the risk of cuts, punctures, or lacerations, and to reduce the risk of injury from chemical or thermal burns.

In healthcare environments, there is often a need for bodily protection from contact with microorganisms.

- Fabric or paper gown: wear to protect yourself from infectious patients; wear to protect patient from possible exposure to microorganisms.
- Plastic apron: wear to reduce contact with bodily secretions and chemicals.
- Overalls: wear when there is a risk of splashing from corrosive materials.

Head, Eye, and Ear Protection

Protection of the head is important in many areas.

- Hairnet or hair cover: wear to prevent contamination from falling hair.
- Hard hat: wear when there is a danger of falling objects.

Eyewear provides the worker or patient with protection from splashes.

- Safety spectacles: wear when there is the risk of eye injury from splashing.
- Goggles: if you wear eyeglasses, wear goggles over them instead of safety spectacles.

Ear protection is necessary when there is a risk of auditory damage.

- Ear plugs: wear to reduce harm from noise.
- Ear muffs: wear when operating loud machinery.

Sharps Management

Sharps are any item that has the possibility to puncture or penetrate. Contaminated sharps have a high risk of transmitting blood-borne diseases. All such items need treatment with care at all times to reduce the possibility of injury or contamination. Sharps containers should be:

- Removed and replaced with a new one when full
- Kept in areas where staff may easily access them
- Kept separate from other containers and be easily seen if transported

Linen Handling

Soiled linen should be handled as little as possible and with minimum agitation to prevent gross microbial contamination of the air and of persons handling the linen. Commercial laundry facilities often use water temperatures of at least 160°F and 50–150 ppm of chlorine bleach to remove significant quantities of microorganisms from grossly contaminated linen.

- All linen should be handled carefully so that there is minimum dispersion of microorganisms.
- Personnel should wear protective equipment when handling linen soiled with bodily substances.
- Used linen should be bagged at the location of use in an appropriate laundry receptacle.
- Linen heavily soiled with blood or other bodily substances should be placed in leak-proof bags and securely tied.
- Hands should be washed after handling used linen.

Vaccination

Healthcare workers may be exposed to certain infections in the course of their work. Vaccines are available to provide some protection to workers in a healthcare setting. In general, vaccines do not guarantee complete protection from disease, and there is potential for adverse effects from receiving a vaccine.

Post Exposure Prophylaxis

In some cases where vaccines do not exists, post exposure prophylaxis is another method of protecting the healthcare worker exposed to a life threatening infectious disease. For example, the viral particles for HIV-AIDS may be precipitated out of the blood through use of an antibody injection if given within 4 hours of a significant exposure.

Surveillance for Emerging Infections

Surveillance is the act of infection investigation using the CDC definitions. Determining an infection requires an Infection Control Practitioner (ICP) to review a patient's chart and see if the patient had the signs and symptoms of an infection. Surveillance traditionally involves significant manual data assessment and entry in order to assess preventative actions such as isolation of patients with an infectious disease.

Isolation

In the healthcare context, isolation refers to various physical measures taken to interrupt nosocomial spread of contagious diseases. There are various forms of isolation, which are applied depending on the type of infection, and the likelihood it can spread via air-born particles, by direct skin contact, or via contact with body fluids.

Outbreak Investigation

When an unusual cluster of illness is noted, infection control teams undertake an investigation to determine whether there is a true outbreak, a pseudo out-break or merely a random fluctuation in the frequency of illness. If a true outbreak is discovered, infection control practitioners try to determine what permitted the outbreak to occur, and to rearrange the conditions to prevent ongoing propagation of the infection.

Body Substance Isolation

Body substance isolation is the practice of isolating all body substances of individuals undergoing medical treatment who might be infected with illnesses in order to reduce the chances of transmitting these illnesses. Body substances include blood, urine, feces, tears, and so on. Types of body substance isolation include but are not limited to hospital gowns, medical gloves, shoe covers, surgical masks, and safety glasses.

Sterilization and Disinfection

Sterilization is a process intended to kill all microorganisms and is the highest level of microbial kill that is possible. Sterilizers may be heat, steam, or liquid chemical. Effectiveness of the sterilizer is determined in three ways. First by the mechanical indicators and gauges on the machine itself, second by the heat sensitive indicators or tape on the sterilizing bag turn color, and thirdly and most importantly is the biological test. With the biological test, a highly heat and chemical resistant microorganism selected as the standard challenge. If the process kills this microorganism, the sterilizer considered effective. To be effective, clean instruments are secured otherwise the debris may form a protective barrier, shielding the microbes from the lethal process. Similarly, extra care provided after sterilization to ensure sterile instruments are not contaminated prior to use.

Disinfection is the use of liquid chemicals on surfaces and at room temperature to kill disease-causing microorganisms. Disinfection is a less effective process than sterilization because it does not kill bacterial endospores.

Chapter Summary

- The United States Pharmacopeia (USP 797) is the official public standards setting authority to safeguard the safeties of all the manufactured drugs.
- Hazardous material is any substance or mixture of substances having properties capable of producing adverse effects on the health and safety or the environment of a human being.
- Proper counting, dispensing, and documentation of controlled substances and investigational drugs is a must.
- Aseptic technique must be observed at all times.
- The selecting, handling, storage, transport, use, and disposal of hazardous materials and wastes are managed through programs located in online HSC Clinical Operations Safety Policies and Procedures and in the online Risk, Safety, Health and Environmental Affairs Manual.
- Radiopharmaceuticals are unique medicinal formulations containing radioisotopes which are used in major clinical areas for diagnosis and/or therapy.
- Infection control policies and procedures are designed to help all the healthcare workers and patients remain free from transmission of infection.
- Standard Precautions are defined as safe work practices for the care and treatment of all patients, regardless of their known or presumed infectious status.
- Laminar flow hoods are used to prevent contamination of semiconductor wafers, biological samples, or any particle-sensitive device.

PRACTICE TEST QUESTIONS

Infection Control and Hazardous Materials

1. The first line of defense in infection control is:

   a. clean apparel
   b. handwashing
   c. private rooms for all patients
   d. none of the above

2. Hazardous drugs are drugs involved in treating cancer. The term(s) used to describe these drugs is:

   a. chemotherapeutic
   b. statins
   c. biguanides
   d. aminoglycosides

3. The definition of *nosocomial infection* is:

   a. an infection caused by an organism that requires a host for nourishment
   b. an infection caused by exposure to a parasite
   c. an infection acquired while hospitalized
   d. an infection acquired by a mosquito bite

4. The type of Laminar Air Hood (LAH) used to prepare cancer medication is:

   a. horizontal
   b. open
   c. vertical
   d. any of these types of hoods are acceptable

5. When handling antineoplastic medications, the technician usually wears how many pairs of gloves?

   a. don't need to wear gloves if the technician is cautious
   b. one pair for all drugs
   c. don't need to wear gloves if the cuff of the protective gown is long
   d. two pair

6. Contact with chemotherapy medications can cause:

   a. dizziness
   b. nausea
   c. skin rash
   d. all of the above

7. When cleaning a laminar airflow hood, the technician must use:

   a. 70% isopropyl alcohol
   b. soap and water
   c. hot water only
   d. any of the above

8. When disposing of sharps, the technician should always clip the needle before placing in the disposal.

   a. true
   b. false

9. ASHP recommends that personnel wash their hands for how long before compounding?

   a. 30 seconds
   b. 15 seconds
   c. 60 seconds
   d. 45 seconds

10. Sterile products should be prepared in a:

    a. Class 50 environment
    b. Class 75 environment
    c. Class 100 environment
    d. Class 200 environment

11. If skin or eye contact to a hazardous drug occurs, the technician should following these steps:

    a. rinse the eye immediately with an eyewash fountain and contact a supervisor
    b. establish first aid and document the injury
    c. obtain medical attention and document the injury
    d. rinse the eye immediately with an eyewash fountain, obtain medical attention and document the injury

12. When disposing of hazardous materials, the technician should:

    a. dispose the material when container is full
    b. dispose the material separately from other trash
    c. dispose the material with other trash
    d. any of the above is appropriate

13. Which of the following is *not* a form of infection transmission in healthcare settings?

    a. airborne transmission
    b. otic transmission
    c. droplet transmission
    d. contact transmission

14. The difference between bactericidal and bacteriostatic agents is:

    a. bactericidal agents prevent the growth of bacteria
    b. bacteriostatic agents kill bacteria
    c. bactericidal agents kill bacteria
    d. bactericidal agents are chemical agents produced by organisms used to treat infection

15. In a hospital pharmacy setting, the process most at risk for contamination is:

    a. handling drugs
    b. liquid preparation
    c. compounding
    d. IV preparation

16. Prior to compounding preparation, the technician needs to clean countertops and equipment with:

a. alcohol
b. water
c. warm soap and water
d. any of the above

17. Laminar flow hoods should be cleaned:

a. once a day
b. at least 30 minutes before using
c. at least 60 minutes before using
d. twice a day

18. Hands should always be washed or sanitized when:

a. before working in an air flow hood
b. entering the IV room
c. before prepare a compounding medication
d. all of the above

19. Which of the skills listed is the *most* important aspect of preparing sterile products?

a. aseptic technique
b. using 70% isopropyl alcohol to wipe down the hood
c. discarding of used needles
d. cleaning the surface with soap and water

20. According to USP 797 regulations, what *should not* be worn during compounding preparation?

a. hair ties
b. gloves
c. artificial nails
d. all of the above

16

Facility Management

Test Topics

After completing this chapter, you should be able to demonstrate knowledge of the following:

1. Storage requirements and expiration dates for equipment and supplies
2. Security systems for the protection of employees, customers, and property
3. Equipment calibration and maintenance procedures
4. Supply procurement procedures
5. Purpose and function of pharmacy equipment
6. Documentation requirements for routine sanitation, maintenance, and equipment calibration
7. Americans with Disabilities Act requirements
8. Downtime emergency policies and procedures

Test Terms

- **aseptic technique** a method used to prevent the contamination of an object by microorganisms
- **crash carts** trays used by all areas of a hospital that contain injectable medications used for a code blue (respiratory distress)
- **ergodynamics** the applied science concerned with designing and arranging equipment and people so that they can work efficiently and safely
- **high-efficiency particulate air (HEPA) filter** a special filter that traps all particles larger than 0.2 µm
- **periodic automatic replenishment level** the minimum amount of medication that a pharmacy should have in stock at any given time

Pharmacy equipment, supplies, and facilities comprise the necessary items that make the practice of pharmacy possible. From corner drugstores to hospitals to long-term care facilities, there are requisite supplies that all pharmacies rely on, and there are standards for the function, care, and maintenance of them. Storing, supplying, and protecting pharmacies is a job unto itself, and oftentimes, the pharmacy technicians are required to do the work that keeps things running smoothly.

In addition to stocking, cleaning, and equipping pharmacies, there are federal laws and guidelines that must be followed regarding the safety and accessibility of pharmacies. Working in hospital or store-chain pharmacies, you may not realize that there are laws that must be adhered to from the parking lot to the restrooms to ensure that everyone has access to care and service. Safety and security of personnel, customers, and patient information are top priority in the pharmacy, and again, pharmacy technicians are relied upon to ensure that standards are met and procedures are followed.

Pharmacy Equipment

Depending on the type of pharmacy that employs you, you will come across different equipment. The equipment that you find in a hospital pharmacy varies greatly from that which is supplied in a community pharmacy. A long-term care facility may require different equipment than a hospital pharmacy as well. Regardless of where you are employed, there are procedures in place to ensure that the equipment is maintained, serviced, and calibrated properly. Much of that information will be found in your pharmacy's policies and procedures manual.

Sterile Product Preparation

Although pharmacy equipment improves the speed and efficiency of processes in the pharmacy, the main purpose of it is accuracy. The practice of pharmacy is precise, and reliable equipment is necessary to ensure that preparations are performed precisely.

Pharmacy technicians who work in settings in which IV, ophthalmic, chemother- apeutic, and parenteral nutrition orders are prepared must know how to use the equipment involved in these preparations properly and safely. In addition, pharmacy technicians are responsible for the maintenance and calibration of pharmacy equip- ment. You will be trained in the effective use of **aseptic technique**, which is a method used to prevent the contamination of an object by microorganisms (see Chapter 9). All pharmacy technicians are tested on the use of aseptic technique, usually yearly, unless there has been a case of contamination, which would require more frequent testing. To test a pharmacy technician's ability, typically a sample of a newly prepared sterile product will be taken and sent to a laboratory to test for microorganism growth.

Equipment and Supplies

Hospital pharmacies perform the widest range of parenteral product preparations. In order to prepare sterile products, there are specific supplies required. An IV preparation room is a standard space in a hospital, and sometimes long-term care, pharmacy. Some of the supplies found in such an IV room include

- *70% isopropyl alcohol* – for cleaning the hood
- *alcohol pads* – convenient for swabbing
- *filter needles* – a filter that prevents gas from entering the final solution when drawing an ampule
- *filter straws* – for pulling medication from ampules
- *filters* – used to trap particulates from entering intravenous fluids
- *male/female adapter* – fits a syringe on each end for mixing two contents
- *syringe needles* – including common bore sizes
- *syringe caps* – sterile cap to prevent the contamination of syringes once they leave the pharmacy
- *syringes* – to hold 0.3 to 60 ml for the administration of medication
- *transfer needles* – a needle on both ends to transfer a vial to a bottle
- *tubing for pumps* – for a specific manufacturer's machine
- *tubing transfer sets* – used to transfer large containers into empty containers
- *mini spike* – large spike that is pushed into a vial with a syringe attachment at the other end
- *forceps* – for closing off tubing while transferring medication

It is the pharmacy technician's duty to ensure that the IV room is stocked properly, so get to know what's expected to be on hand in the IV room at your facility. Before and after each shift, you should reorder and restock the supplies for the next shift. The time for stock to arrive can range from a few hours to up to a week, depend- ing on whether the supplies are being sent from the centralized pharmacy or from an off-site manufacturer, so be aware of what supplies may take longer to be in hand so that the IV room is always fully stocked.

Horizontal flow hoods are used for many types of parenteral medication preparations and sterile product mixtures. In this type of hood, the outside air flows into the back of the hood, through a **high-efficiency particulate air (HEPA)** filter, and then out toward the opening. Air direction moves from the back of the hood to the front. Because the sides of the hood and items within it create a disruption of airflow, you must work 6 inches from the sides and front of the hood.

Vertical flow hoods are used specifically for the preparation of chemotherapeutic agents because of the direction of the airflow. Air direction flows from the top of the hood to the bottom. The airflow is similar to that of the horizontal flow hood except that the air cannot reenter the room. Therefore, vertical hoods have a Plexiglas shield that separates the pharmacy technician from the inside work surface. The vertical flow hood has two HEPA filters in place: the first filters the air that comes into the workspace area, and the second filters the air before it is released into the room or is vented outside.

Equipment Calibration and Maintenance

Pharmacy equipment generally has an expiration date of one year. This means that within a year's time, an authorized inspector should verify that the equipment is still functioning effectively, efficiently, and accurately. Laminar flow hoods are inspected yearly by an authorized inspector to ensure that the filtering system is working effectively. HEPA filters should be inspected every 6 months and have their prefilters changed frequently.

Compounding equipment, such as syringe pumps and automated total parenteral nutrition compounders, should be inspected, calibrated, and maintained according to the manufacturer's instructions.

Balances are often used to measure powder, liquid, and viscous agents for compounding purposes. Many balances are digital and self-calibrating. However, some pharmacies still use weighted balances that require manual calibration. This task falls to the pharmacy technician. When calibrating a balance, you must first place the weights to the right side of the balance. This will ensure that you return the most accurate reading. If you're unsure of whether a balance is accurately calibrated, you may calibrate the balance again, ask another pharmacy technician to assist you, or check with a pharmacist on duty.

Sanitation of Equipment

Maintaining sterile equipment is essential to ensuring that sterile products are free from contaminating microorganisms. Follow the instructions carefully for the cleaning of Laminar flow hoods in particular. The proper procedures for garbing and gloving in a sterile environment should be provided by the facility in which you work, and you will be evaluated regularly on your garbing and gloving habits.

Cleaning the horizontal hood should occur at the beginning of the day and periodically throughout the day to ensure a sterile environment. Follow these steps:

- Remove materials from inside the hood.
- Don the appropriate gown, gloves, and other protective outerwear.
- Moisten 4 × 4-inch gauze or other disposable cloth with 70% isopropyl alcohol and wet down the inside of the hood.
- Starting at the top right-hand side, wipe down, across the surface, and up to the top of the left-hand side of the hood.
- Repeat the motion in the opposite direction.
- Don't go back over what has already been cleaned. Cleaning is done in one direction from top to bottom on the sides and from back to top on the table surface.

Cleaning the vertical hood should also occur at the beginning of the day and then periodically throughout the day to ensure a sterile environment. Follow these steps:

- Moisten 4 × 4-inch gauze or other disposable cloth with 70% isopropyl alcohol and wipe down the inside of the hood, including the back, sides, and tabletop; do NOT spray the ceiling.
- Start on the inside back of the hood and wipe from the top right across to the left-hand side, drop down a few inches, and then back across to the other side, continuing in this way until the back wall is completed.
- Repeat from the top right-hand side, across the tabletop, and up the other side until the entire hood is completed.
- Wash down the inside of the Plexiglas protective shield last.

> **RECALL TIP**
>
> When cleaning the hood, imagine that you are painting a picture with the alcohol-soaked gauze, covering every centimeter of the hood in the methodical way. Not missing a speck of space will ensure a sterile environment for the next sterile preparation.

Documentation Requirements

Hospitals, especially those certified by the JCAHO, require that maintenance, calibration, and sterilization of equipment are documented for their annual audits. This documentation is crucial, especially if there is a case of contamination, the source of which can often be pinpointed by evaluating the documentation kept at the facility.

Drug storage refrigerators require daily monitoring and documentation to ensure temperatures between 36 and 46°F. Some refrigerators can be fitted with an alarm that will sound if the temperature falls outside of a preset range. Temperatures can be documented in a log book, journal, or electronically in a stored system, depending on the preference of the facility.

There should be monthly inspection of all drug storage locations by pharmacy technicians. This inspection should ensure:

- Compliance with appropriate storage conditions
- Separation of drugs and food
- Proper use of multidose vials
- Avoidance of single-dose vials being used as multidose vials
- Proper storage of compounded sterile products away from unauthorized personnel, visitors, and patients

Equipment, including chairs, tables, and flooring, should be made of materials that are easily cleaned and disinfected. Equipment should be maintained on a schedule and documented according to the policies and procedures of the facility.

Supply Procurement

Pharmacies rely on their stock to meet the daily prescription needs for their patients and customers. Effective treatment, especially in hospitals where patients are beholden to the in-house pharmacy to provide their medication, relies on a well-stocked pharmacy. Pharmacy technicians are expected to maintain the stock levels of medications at their facilities, and there are many responsibilities that come with this job.

Ordering Systems

How do pharmacies maintain their stock of medications and supplies? Most pharmacies rely on their pharmacy technicians to ensure that an adequate supply of medications is kept on hand. The established level of medication stock kept on hand at any given time is known as the **periodic automatic replenishment level**. This is the *minimum* amount of medication that a pharmacy should have in stock at any given time. There are many types of systems to keep a running inventory of medications and order them, including:

- at the point of sale
- using order cards
- using handheld inventory computers

Pharmacy technicians are in charge of all aspects of ordering, restocking, and returning stock within the pharmacy, so it is helpful to be familiar with different ordering systems. Most pharmacies use computerized systems to monitor their stock levels. Let's take a look at some of the types of ordering systems available.

Bar Coding

Most products are identifiable via bar codes that can be scanned. At the very least, these unique codes tag the drug's:

- name
- strength
- dosage form
- quantity
- cost
- package size

Pharmacies can use these bar codes to track their stock level at the register (point-of-sale). When the item is scanned, it is automatically removed from the computerized inventory list. When the in-stock quantity falls to the periodic automatic replenishment level, it is automatically reordered. Bar codes can also be used with handheld ordering devices, wherein the pharmacy technician scans the medication with the device and enters the quantity desired. The information that the handheld device gathers is then sent to the main computer ordering system.

Automated Dispensing Systems

Some hospitals have multiple pharmacies within them, including satellite pharmacies, drug cabinets, and drug carts that are located throughout the facility. How can the stock level be determined when the medication is away from the shelf? Automated dispensing systems link the nursing units to the pharmacy computer system so that real-time stock information can be viewed at any time. When a nurse enters the type and amount of drug removed from a drug cabinet, the inventory level in that drug cabinet is automatically adjusted, and that information is passed along to the pharmacy's main database. Reports can be obtained for stock levels of a specific medication throughout the hospital from one centralized computer. This computer can also monitor controlled substance use and inventory, keeping a log for all users.

In community pharmacies, similar automated systems are used. The Baker cell system keeps track of inventory as tablets and capsules are dispensed into drug vials. As each pill passes through a beam of light, it is removed from the pharmacy's inventory.

Manual Ordering

Despite the uptick in computerized ordering systems, many pharmacies rely on manually monitored drug levels. Pharmacy technicians note that a drug's stock is getting low, and they may use ordering cards that stay inside the medication box which list the drug information, ordering number, and the periodic automatic replenishment levels to give a reference for the technician to order the right amount. Either the card

RECALL TIP

Preparing a manual medication order in a busy pharmacy setting can easily get interrupted by ringing phones, lines of customers, and prescriptions to be filled. To keep from skipping medications in the order when you get a chance to pick back up, grab a bottle of the medication you are in the process of ordering and set it aside with your order book. This will take you right back to where you left off when you return the stock bottle to the shelf.

system or simply writing down the right amount of stock to be ordered depends on the pharmacy technician's knowledge of the drug's category:

- *Formulary* – an organized list of drugs approved by the P & T Committee for use in an institution or by a prescription drug benefit plan
- *Nonformulary* – fewer nonformulary drugs are kept on hand because they're prescribed less frequently
- *Fast mover* – high-volume use drugs, kept separate from the regular stock, ordered in large quantities and ordered often
- *Slow mover* – not commonly prescribed except by a few doctors, their expiration dates should be checked frequently
- *Special order* – usually ordered at time of use, only used by a few patients
- *Time of year* – some medications are fast movers only at certain times of the year, so their stock levels need periodic adjustment

It takes time to become familiar with the medications that are prescribed more frequently in your particular pharmacy, so be aware of physicians and their prescribing habits, and take note of the change of seasons to have ample supply of things like asthma inhalers, allergy medicine, and antibiotic suspensions for children when the time comes.

Checking in Stock

When medication arrives from a warehouse or off-site facility, it will come with a packing slip and invoice that needs to be verified against what was shipped to the pharmacy. Follow these steps to check in medications from a stock order:

- Obtain the warehouse invoice.
- Verify that the number of boxes shipped is equal to the number of boxes received.
- Refrigerate or freeze medications that are marked as such immediately.
- For each product, check against the invoice for the drug name, strength, dosage form, quantity, and expiration date.
- Compare the invoice with the order form to make sure that only what was ordered was received.
- Sign and date the invoice and send it for processing according to your pharmacy's procedures.
- Begin to put the stock away, rotating the new stock behind the current stock to keep expiration dates in order.
- If manually ordered, return the inventory cards to the medication box for future use.

Storing the medications in their proper place is important. Refrigerated, light-protected, or frozen items must be stored as soon as possible in the proper location. Some chemicals must be kept behind cabinet doors because they are toxic. Follow the maufacturer's guidelines for the proper storage of medications and supplies to ensure that the items are not rendered unusable.

Returning Medication

Medications can be sent back to the manufacturer for three primary reasons:

- Drug recalls
- Damaged stock
- Expired stock

Each pharmacy's policies and procedures manual will cover the steps to take when returning medicine. However, this task usually falls to the pharmacy technician, so you need to be familiar with why and how to return medicine.

Drug Recalls

Occasionally the U.S. Food and Drug Administration (FDA) will find cause to recall a medication from the market, and by law, the medication must be returned. These reasons may include:

- Incorrect labeling of the medication
- Improper packaging or production of the product
- Contaminated drug batch
- Other changes that cause the drug to fall outside of the FDA's or manufacturer's guidelines

The FDA will emit the recall information by postal mail or by fax, and the procedure to be followed for responding to the recall will be outlined in the directive. The lot number of the drug will be included on the correspondence, and this is the key piece of information in identifying the drug to be returned. The pharmacy technician will check the stock to determine whether the particular drug is in stock; if it is not, then you initial the recall form to indicate that it is not stocked. If the drug is in stock, then a pharmacist must be alerted so that any patients who had received that medication can be contacted by phone about the recalled drug or device.

FDA prefers that the manufacturer voluntarily recalls a drug. All recalled products must be returned to the manufacturer as they prescribe. If this depletes your pharmacy's stock of a drug, then new stock of that drug must be ordered immediately, perhaps from another manufacturer or supplier.

RECALL TIP
Drug recalls are serious business, and the FDA expects you to react quickly and efficiently when determining whether your stock is affected by a recall. Remember the four R's of a recall: revisit the stock, recheck the lot number, ring the patients who received it, and return the medication to the manufacturer.

Damaged Stock

Some stock may arrive damaged in a shipment from a warehouse or other supplier. If you failed to notice this before checking in and signing off on an invoice, you can still return the drug to the manufacturer. Usually calling the manufacturer or supplier first to receive an approval code for the return is the best course of action so that they can reference your return for receipt and send out a replacement quickly.

Expired Stock

Pharmacies often have a policy of pulling drugs from stock that have an expiration date of three months or sooner so that there are no drugs on the shelves that are on the brink of expiration. Sending expired medications in batches of multiple bottles is more efficient than sending one or two bottles every week. Follow the manufacturer's guidelines for the return of expired medication and other items. Hazardous chemicals must be handled especially carefully so that they do not break open or leak during transport.

Nonreturnable Stock

There are plenty of items that manufacturers will not accept back, so what do you do with them? Repackaged medications, reconstituted medications, and partial bottles are examples of items that a manufacturer will not accept for credit. Many of these items can be disposed of in the pharmacy's garbage, but some chain pharmacies prefer that the drugs be sent to a centralized location for their destruction or return for credit.

Some hazardous items, such as cytotoxic agents, must be disposed of in sharps containers indicating hazardous waste. Nontoxic intravenous agents are disposed of in regular sharps containers. Controlled substances must be counted and cosigned by a pharmacist before they are destroyed. Contact the DEA before disposing of any scheduled medications, because they have certain policies and procedures for that task. The DEA issues a receipt for schedule II merchandise that is destroyed, and that receipt must be retained by the pharmacy for five years with the schedule II inventory (see Chapter 15).

Supplying Departmental Needs

Each department in a hospital has its own set of typical medications that need to be stocked depending on the types of service it provides. For example, a labor and delivery floor stock will contain medications pertaining to labor, contractions, and Caesarean births, whereas a pediatric unit might have mostly suspension-form or lower-dose medications. The tasks of supplying and stocking these floor stock medications fall to the pharmacy technician under the guidance and approval of a pharmacist.

Crash carts, which are trays used by all areas of the hospital, contain injectable medications that are used for a code blue (respiratory distress). Pharmacy technicians are responsible for refilling the crash carts throughout the hospital. The central pharmacy stocks trays that are prepared in advance in the case of an emergency call for a crash cart. There are three types of trays containing a different strength of drug:

- adult
- pediatric
- neonatal

Crash carts contain a security lock which is broken when the tray is brought into use. The pharmacy technician refills the used tray with the missing contents and checks the expiration dates of the medications. It is important that you place the medications on the tray in the same order each time, since precious seconds can mean the difference between life and death if a nurse or doctor has to search the tray's medication for the one that should be in his or her reach. All orders are verified by the pharmacist before the tray is secured and returned to the correct departments.

Accessibility and Security

Pharmacies and hospitals are public settings whose structures and layouts are governed by guidelines and laws set forth by the federal government and other agencies. The U.S. population consists of people with various degrees of limitations and accessibility issues that must be accommodated by law. In addition, the hospitals and pharmacies must ensure the safety of the personnel and patients who cross their thresholds each day, as well as the personal data with which they're entrusted. One way pharmacies protect their patients is by allowing only authorized personnel into the pharmacy area.

Accessibility

RECALL TIP

The Americans with Disabilities Act of 1990 protects people with disabilities from bias and discrimination. You may find yourself in situations where a person with a disability requires assistance that can only come from a person. Help them reach something on a shelf, pick up something they've dropped, read the information on their prescription bag, or wrangle their overcoat. Helping others in their time of need goes a long way to extending the care and concern that should be synonymous with healthcare personnel.

Public access to public buildings is considered a civil right based on the Americans with Disabilities Act of 1990. According to this law, it is illegal to prohibit the civil rights of anyone based on a disability. There are several tiers to the law that covers all areas of life in the United States, but Title III, which covers public accommodations and commercial facilities, describes that no one can be disallowed access to public accommodations because of a disability. Examples of these include:

- hotels
- recreation
- transportation
- education
- dining
- stores
- care providers, including hospitals and pharmacies

Pharmacies and hospitals must provide access to their services to all people. Therefore, the aisles must be wide enough to accommodate a wheelchair, the counter must be low enough for a patient in a wheelchair to see and communicate with pharmacy personnel, the parking lot must have handicap-accessible spaces and ramps, and you may be asked to assist a person with any accessibility needs they may have while in your facility.

Workplace Safety

Safety guidelines are important to follow to ensure that the personnel, customers, and patients remain free of harm. The United States Department of Labor's Occupational Safety and Health Administration (OSHA) is responsible for setting forth and enforcing the implementation of safety standards in the workplace. OSHA's purpose is to help prevent work-related injuries and illnesses.

OSHA Guidelines

You can thank OSHA for the regulations surrounding personal protective equipment, such as goggles, gloves, coveralls, and so forth when handling hazardous materials. Countless infections and high-risk situations have been avoided thanks to their standards of operations. One of their most readily recognizable guidelines is that surrounding **ergodynamics**, which is the applied science concerned with designing and arranging equipment and people so that they can work efficiently and safely. These guidelines apply to such things as:

- computer terminal placement
- chairs
- placement of furniture
- keyboards
- telephones
- lighting

Pharmacies and hospitals are required to follow OSHA guidelines to improve the safety of the workplace for everyone. If you have an issue with any OSHA-regulated areas of your facility, bring it to the immediate attention of your pharmacy manager.

Fire Safety

Depending on the type of pharmacy in which you work, the fire exits may be located in various places. If you're in a centralized pharmacy in the basement of a hospital, for instance, your exits may be different from those in a storefront pharmacy in a downtown retail chain. At minimum, there must be two fire exits in any pharmacy.

Portable fire extinguishers should be located in every pharmacy as well, and all personnel should be trained on their use. Because you will have contact with various types of flammable agents, you must be certain that the correct fire extinguisher is used in an emergency situation. Otherwise, the wrong choice could spread the fire and make matters worse. There are four classes of fire extinguishers:

- Class A – for ordinary combustibles, such as wood, cloth, and paper
- Class B – for fires involving flammable agents such as liquids, greases, and gasses
- Class C – for fires involving energized electrical equipment
- Class D – for fires involving metals such as titanium, magnesium, zirconium, sodium, and potassium

In addition, letter-shaped symbol markings are also used to indicate extinguisher suitability according to the class of fire:

- Class A – green triangle containing the letter A
- Class B – red square containing the letter B

- Class C – blue circle containing the letter C
- Class D – five-pointed star containing the letter D

The National Fire Protection Association (NFPA) affixes a diamond atop each portable fire extinguisher that is broken into four colored (red, yellow, blue, and white) smaller diamond quadrants. Numbers in the three colored diamonds range from 0 (least severe hazard) to 4 (most severe hazard). The fourth (white) diamond is left blank and is only used to denote special fire-fighting measures or hazards. The information relayed via the diamonds is primarily for firefighters and other emergency responders, but a familiarity with the system is important for anyone in a position to use a fire extinguisher. The colors indicate:

- Blue diamond – health hazard
- Red diamond – flammability
- Yellow diamond – instability
- White diamond – special hazards

Personal Security

Pharmacies are targets for crimes of all types: forged prescriptions, robberies for cash, robberies for controlled substances, retaliatory crimes as a result of service or health issues. Steps are taken to ensure the safety of personnel as well as customers in the pharmacy, and the policies and procedures manual outlines those facility-specific steps that have been taken on your behalf. As a customer, you may notice things in your local community pharmacy that are security measures, such as:

- Protective glass fronting the pharmacy
- Security cameras monitoring the parking lot, front and rear doors, and pharmacy fill area
- Counseling areas set apart from pickup and drop-off windows
- Security guards patrolling the store
- Locked-door or keycard access to the pharmacy fill area

In addition to physical security measures, pharmacy technicians receive a user name and password for access to the pharmacy's computer system to keep their computer use protected. This protects the personal information of patients and records, and it provides a tracking system to determine what personnel may have accessed information or processed certain prescriptions during a particular time period. This system ensures accountability, and the work done at a particular workstation is backed up daily onto the facility's computer mainframe. For your own safety and accountability, do not share your password with anyone, and when prompted, change it to something only you would know.

Chapter Summary

- Pharmacy equipment improves the accuracy of work accomplished in the pharmacy.
- IV, ophthalmic, chemotherapeutic, and parenteral nutrition orders are prepared using aseptic techniques.
- Isopropyl alcohol is primarily used for the sterilization of pharmacy equipment.
- A pharmacy's IV room is stocked and maintained by the pharmacy technician.
- Laminar flow hoods are used for the preparation of sterile products.
- Vertical flow hoods are specifically used for the preparation of chemotherapeutic agents.

- Pharmacy equipment is evaluated yearly by a certified professional inspector.
- Cleaning the Laminar flow hoods should be done throughout the day to ensure a sterile environment with each use.
- Monitoring and documentation guidelines are outlined by manufacturers and by the facility's policies and procedures manual.
- Pharmacy technicians can order supplies via point of sale, order cards, or inventory computers.
- Checking in stock against the invoice ensures that all medications are accounted for and none is damaged.
- Checking in refrigerated, frozen, or light-protected items first ensures their proper storage and reduces spoilage.
- Drug recalls are regulated by the FDA and must be followed.
- Crash cart replenishment is the duty of the pharmacy technician and requires attention to detail.
- The Americans with Disabilities Act of 1990 ensures unrestricted access to all citizens regardless of disability.
- OSHA guidelines enforce safety standards in the workplace, including ergodynamic work spaces.
- At least two fire exits should exist in every pharmacy.
- Fire extinguishers contain codes that identify the types of fires they are suitable for extinguishing.
- Safety measures within the pharmacy are taken to keep personnel safe from personal and environmental threats.
- Using a password when accessing a pharmacy computer ensures your accountability and protects the patient files contained within the system.

PRACTICE TEST QUESTIONS

Facility Management

1. What duties should a pharmacy technician perform in anticipation of the day in the pharmacy?
   a. make sure the IV clean room is stocked
   b. turn on equipment that will be used throughout the day
   c. turn on Laminar air flow hoods
   d. all of the above

2. The applied science concerned with designing and arranging the equipment personnel use so they can work efficiently and safely is called:
   a. JCAHO compliance
   b. ergonomics
   c. OSHA compliance
   d. Economics

3. How many exits must be designated as fire exits in a pharmacy?
   a. one
   b. three
   c. two
   d. four

4. What class of first extinguisher is used for flammable agents?
   a. Class A
   b. Class B
   c. Class C
   d. Class D

5. Which organization is responsible for making sure pharmacies follow safety guidelines?
   a. OSHA
   b. JCAHO
   c. FDA
   d. DEA

6. A security system that protects pharmacy personnel as well as customers is:
   a. cameras
   b. a common password for only pharmacy personnel

c. protective glass for pharmacy personnel
d. all of the above

7. The pharmacy personnel responsible for calibrating and maintaining pharmacy equipment is the:

   a. pharmacy manager
   b. pharmacist in charge
   c. pharmacy technician
   d. building maintenance

8. Pharmacy equipment should have an expiration date of:

   a. six months
   b. one year
   c. two years
   d. three years

9. The *main* purpose of pharmacy equipment is:

   a. accuracy
   b. making the work easier
   c. speed
   d. less cleanup

10. When calibrating the accuracy of a balance, the weights should always be placed on which side of the balance?

    a. left
    b. either
    c. right
    d. combination

11. If a pharmacy technician is unsure about the calibration of a balance, he or she should:

    a. recheck the calibration
    b. consult another technician
    c. consult a pharmacist
    d. any of the above

12. When prepare a compounding medication, a pharmacy technician should clean all equipment with:

    a. warm water
    b. alcohol
    c. soap and water
    d. hot water

13. One of the responsibilities of a hospital technician is the stocking of a crash cart. How does a technician determine whether the cart needs to be restocked?

    a. the pharmacist informs the technician
    b. the nurse informs the technician
    c. the security lock is broken
    d. the technician checks for missing medications daily

14. The red portion of the diamond-shaped warning label on a fire extinguisher signifies:

    a. flammability
    b. health hazards
    c. instability
    d. special hazards

15. The blue portion of the diamond-shaped warning label on a fire extinguisher signifies:

    a. flammability
    b. health hazards
    c. instability
    d. special hazards

16. When using the computer to protect against possible abusers or to record a pharmacy personnel's activities, each authorized person is issued a:

    a. key to turn the computer on
    b. user ID that includes their first initial and last name
    c. password
    d. number

17. Every computer system has a database of information. These files must be:

    a. kept separate
    b. backed up daily
    c. kept in alphabetical order
    d. kept in an operation manual

18. Some drugs must be stored at a constant temperature. If refrigerated, the temperature should be recorded daily and logged generally between:

    a. 22–29°F
    b. 27–32°F
    c. 32–38°F
    d. 36–46°F

19. A logbook is one way to document routine equipment requirements.

    a. true
    b. false

20. The Americans with Disabilities Act requirements pharmacies to accommodate the disabled by:

    a. providing wheelchair ramps
    b. providing accessible aisles for travel
    c. parking accommodations
    d. all of the above

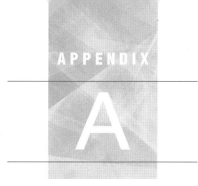

APPENDIX

A

Answers to Chapter Practice Test Questions

Chapter 2: Law and Ethics

1. Which amendment or act is also known as the prescription drug amendment?
   a. Kefauver-Harris Amendment
   b. Omnibus Budget Reconciliation Act
   c. Durham-Humphrey Amendment
   d. Poison Prevention Packaging Act

2. Which of the following is considered "confidential" information?
   a. Directory information
   b. License number
   c. Country of origin
   d. Marital status

3. Which organization enforces the Poison Prevention Packaging Act?
   a. The Council of Health-System Pharmacists
   b. Food and Drug Administration
   c. Drug Enforcement Administration
   d. Consumer Product Safety Commission

4. What is a safe and effective drug?
   a. A medication classified as a Schedule V controlled substance
   b. A drug approved by the FDA for sale in the United States
   c. A medication that prevents pregnancy
   d. A drug that has no side effects

5. The Kefauver-Harris Amendment of 1962 requires drug manufacturers prove to the FDA:
   a. the effectiveness of their products before marketing them.
   b. that household substances packaged for consumers use child-resistant packaging.
   c. that drugs which cannot be used safely without medical supervision, be labeled for sale and be dispensed by a prescription of an authorized prescriber.
   d. All of the above

6. When completing DEA form 222 to obtain Schedule II medications, which requirement must be met?
   a. Copies one and two must be forwarded to the wholesaler, with the carbon paper intact.
   b. The form must be handwritten in pencil.
   c. More than one item must be ordered per line.
   d. Suppliers must accept and fill an order even if it has errors and erasures.

7. Which federal law ensured that drugs being distributed were safe and fulfilled reported claims?
   a. Controlled Substances Act
   b. Omnibus Budget Reconciliation Act
   c. Food, Drug, and Cosmetic Act
   d. Durham-Humphrey Act

8. Which law requires pharmacists to counsel patients on new medications?
   a. Durham-Humphrey's Amendment
   b. Comprehensive Drug Abuse Prevention and Control Act
   c. Prescription Drug Marketing Act
   d. Omnibus Budget Reconciliation Act

9. What is the purpose of the Orphan Drug Act?
   a. Stops the use of drugs without a prescription in animals
   b. Allows drug companies to bypass lengthy testing to treat persons who have a rare disease
   c. Ensures safety and effectiveness of manufacturing practices
   d. Applies stricter rules concerning controlled substances sales and distribution

10. The best time to check for errors on a prescription while filling is:
    a. when the order is first received, during filling, and after filling.
    b. while filling the order, after filling, and when handing the medication to the patient.
    c. when checking the original order against the label, against the stock bottle before filling, and before filling the vial and labeling.
    d. before applying the label, before applying the auxiliary labels, and before giving the final product to the pharmacist to check.

11. Which of the following statements identifies "blanket consent"?
    a. A separate consent form must be signed for each individual procedure.
    b. The consent outlines many items of routine care and/or information and is signed on the first encounter with a healthcare provider.
    c. The physician regarding risks, side effects and benefits must be given detailed information.
    d. It is used in case of emergency.

12. The middle segment of a national drug code represents which of the following product elements?
    a. **Product code, strength, and dosage form**
    b. Package size, manufacturer, and strength
    c. Dosage form and manufacturer
    d. Package size and product strength

13. In a court of law, the intentional altering of records will result in a charge of:
    a. felony.
    b. misdemeanor.
    c. forgery.
    d. fraud.

14. The Patient Self-Determination Act, a federal law relating to end-of-life decisions for patients with terminal illnesses, requires two different documents under federal law. The two documents are called:
    a. Emergency Consent and Durable Power of Attorney.
    b. Advance Directive and Specific Consent.
    c. **Durable Power of Attorney and Living Will**
    d. General Consent and Guardian Directive.

15. Which of the following statements about transfer requirements is TRUE regarding refillable non-controlled substances?
    a. Prescriptions can be refilled three times between non-related, non-networked pharmacies.
    b. **Prescriptions can be refilled as many times as the prescription is refillable if the pharmacies share an electronic real-time database.**
    c. Prescriptions can be refilled as often as the patient and prescriber agree.
    d. Prescription refills are up to the discretion of the pharmacist.

16. Controlled substances for office use can be obtained by a prescriber:
    a. **through DEA order form 222.**
    b. with a prescription marked "For Office Use Only."
    c. per a phone order.
    d. by visiting a pharmacy and showing proper identification.

17. A controlled substance inventory must be conducted by a pharmacy:
    a. every year.
    b. **every two years.**
    c. every three years.
    d. every four years.

18. What action can be taken by the DEA if it feels a pharmacy has violated CSA or DEA regulations?
    a. It may seek criminal penalties.
    b. It may seek civil monetary fines.
    c. It may revoke, suspend, or deny the pharmacy's controlled substances registration.
    d. **All of the above**

19. Which statement below is TRUE regarding the Controlled Substances Act?
    a. The Act establishes a system of schedules classifying drugs by their potential for abuse.
    b. The Act requires the registration of individuals and organizations that handle controlled substances.

c. The Act requires strict recordkeeping of controlled substances inventories.
d. **All of the above**

21. A physician prescribes Percocet for a patient going home after abdominal surgery. The patient eventually runs out of the drug and calls the pharmacy for a refill. The technician explains to the patient that:
    a. This medication can only be filled twice.
    b. This medication has an unlimited amount of refills.
    c. **This medication will need another prescription from the physician, because it does not allow refills.**
    d. This medication must be refilled within 30 days of the first prescription.

22. Schedule IV controlled substances can be refilled:
    a. As many times as the provider allows.
    b. **5 times in 6 months.**
    c. Twice.
    d. Zero times; refills are not allowed.

Chapter 3: Medical Abbreviations and Terminology

1. Liquids that carry the direction "Shake Well" are usually:
   a. elixirs.
   b. syrups.
   c. solutions.
   d. **suspensions.**

2. A semisolid dosage form whose base contains more water and penetrates well into the skin are:
   a. creams.
   b. ointments.
   c. **lotions.**
   d. emulsions.

3. A type of dosage form that has a sugar-based solution that the medication dissolves into is called a(n):
   a. elixir.
   b. **syrup.**
   c. aerosol.
   d. suspension.

4. A types of dosage form composed of a gelatin container and comes in different sizes is called a:
   a. caplet.
   b. lozenge.
   c. troche.
   d. **capsule.**

5. A type of liquid dosage form that contains dissolved medication in an alcohol base or water is called a(n):
   a. **elixir.**
   b. syrup.
   c. suspension.
   d. solution.

6. The brand name for glimepiride is:
   a. Actos.
   b. **Amaryl.**
   c. Avandia.
   d. Orinase.

7. Potentiation:
   a. describes a side effect.
   b. is the joint action of a drug.
   c. increases the effect of another drug.
   d. causes a therapeutic effect.

8. The medical abbreviation for 4 times a day is:
   a. QID.
   b. BID.
   c. TID.
   d. QD.

9. The generic name for Azmacort is:
   a. cetirizine.
   b. triamcinolone acetonide.
   c. levalbuterol.
   d. beclomethasone.

10. Decongestants are prescribed to:
    a. treat allergic rhinitis.
    b. eliminate airway obstruction.
    c. treat asthma.
    d. decrease mucous production

11. Theophylline is classified as a(n):
    a. antihistamine.
    b. anticholinergic.
    c. beta 2 agonist.
    d. bronchodilator.

12. The element from the diet that is used by the body to produce thyroid hormone is:
    a. aluminum.
    b. sodium.
    c. iodine.
    d. calcium.

13. The generic name for SoluMedrol is:
    a. methylprednisolone.
    b. prednisone.
    c. prednisolone.
    d. betamethasone.

14. Deltasone, Cortef, and Pediapred are classified as:
    a. Therapeutic corticosteroids.
    b. Hormones to treat osteoporosis.
    c. Glucocorticoids.
    d. Thyroid replacement.

15. All the following are brand names of synthetic levothyroxine except:
    a. Levoxyl.
    b. Cytomel.
    c. Levothroid.
    d. Synthroid.

16. The drug used to treat reversible spasticity or spinal cord lesions is:
    a. tizanadine.
    b. diazepam.
    c. baclofen.
    d. orphenadrine.

17. The neurotransmitter involved with sleep and emotional arousal is:
    a. acetylcholine.
    b. dopamine.

c. norephinephrine.
d. serotonin.

18. The brand name for methocarbamol is:
    a. Dantrium.
    b. Robaxin.
    c. Flexeril.
    d. Zanaflex.

19. What drug is considered to be the "best" muscle relaxer?
    a. Soma
    b. Valium
    c. Lioresal
    d. Flexeril

20. The generic name for Norflex is:
    a. chlorzoxazone.
    b. carisoprodol.
    c. orphenadrine.
    d. baclofen.

21. Pseudoephedrine, phenylephrine, and oxymetolazine are classified as:
    a. alpha adrenergic drugs.
    b. beta adrenergic drugs.
    c. alpha cholinergic drugs.
    d. muscle relaxants.

22. All of the following are drugs used to treat diabetes *except*:
    a. Metformin.
    b. Glipizide.
    c. Glucagon.
    d. HCTZ.

23. The medical abbreviation for after meals is:
    a. AC.
    b. HS.
    c. PO.
    d. PC.

24. The generic name for Allegra is:
    a. oxymetazoline.
    b. fenxofenadine.
    c. clemastine.
    d. trimeprazine.

25. The generic name for Neurontin is:
    a. topiramate.
    b. gabapentin.
    c. carbamazepine.
    d. ethosuximide.

26. The generic name for Inderal is:
    a. benzonatate.
    b. diphenhydramine.
    c. propranolol.
    d. metoclopramide.

27. Tegretol and Zarontin are classified as:
    a. seizure medications.
    b. blocking agents for the reuptake of DA.
    c. anticholinergic agents.
    d. immunosuppressants.

28. The medical abbreviation "ac" means:
    a. after meals.
    b. bedtime.

c. as needed.

d. **before meals.**

29. The generic name for Tensilon is:
    a. methylphenidate.
    b. **edrophonium.**
    c. pyridostigmine.
    d. bromocriptine.

Chapter 4: Anatomy, Physiology, and Disease

1. Asthma primarily affects which part of the lungs?
   a. the alveoli
   b. the air sac
   c. the lung tissue
   d. **the bronchial tubes**

2. Alzheimer disease is a disorder resulting from low levels of the neurotransmitter:
   a. serotonin.
   b. dopamine.
   c. **acetycholine.**
   d. ephinephrine.

3. The adrenal glands are located on the:
   a. liver.
   b. **kidney.**
   c. thyroid.
   d. spleen.

4. The "master gland" of the endocrine system is the:
   a. adrenal gland.
   b. pineal gland.
   c. hypothalamus.
   d. **pituitary gland.**

5. A _____ fracture occurs during the course of normal activity due to osteoporosis.
   a. **stress**
   b. simple
   c. complex
   d. compound

6. The central nervous system consists of the:
   a. **brain and spinal cord.**
   b. brain and autonomic nervous system.
   c. spinal cord and somatic nervous system.
   d. somatic and autonomic nervous systems.

7. In emphysema, there is permanent enlargement of the:
   a. bronchi.
   b. **alveoli.**
   c. bronchioles.
   d. smooth muscle of the lungs.

8. Muscles that control movement such as walking or talking are controlled by the:
   a. autonomic nervous system.
   b. central nervous system.
   c. **somatic nervous system.**
   d. sympathetic nervous system.

9. Neurons that release the neurotransmitter norepinephrine, are referred to as:
   a. affectors.
   b. cholinergic.
   c. effectors.
   d. **adrenergic.**

10. The part of the brain directly involved in the control of many of the body's activities is the:
    a. cerebrum.
    b. cerebellum.
    c. **hypothalamus.**
    d. medulla oblongata.

11. The _____ of the peripheral nervous system are responsible for providing sensory information to the central nervous system.
    a. interneurons
    b. motor neurons
    c. efferent neurons
    d. **afferent neurons**

12. A relatively slow heart rate of less than 60 beats/minute is referred to as:
    a. **bradycardia.**
    b. tachycardia.
    c. sinus arrhythmia.
    d. congestive heart failure.

13. When calculating PTT time, the normal range runs:
    a. 5–10 sec
    b. 10–15 sec
    c. 15–20 sec
    d. **21–35**

14. A patient retaining excessive fluid, resulting in swollen legs and ankles, is likely suffering from:
    a. stroke.
    b. arrhythmia.
    c. **congestive heart failure.**
    d. coronary artery disease.

15. Newly oxygenated blood returning from the lungs enters the heart through which chamber?
    a. **left atrium**
    b. right atrium
    c. left ventricle
    d. right ventricle

16. The main organ of the integumentary system is the:
    a. heart.
    b. lungs.
    c. kidneys.
    d. **skin.**

17. The most common risk factor associated with the development of skin cancer is:
    a. diet.
    b. smoking.
    c. **sun exposure.**
    d. inflammation.

18. The term *onychomycosis* is associated with:
    a. eczema.
    b. skin cancer.
    c. yeast infection.
    d. **fungal infection of the nail beds.**

19. Drugs prescribed to relax the smooth muscles of the arteries, the prostate, and the bladder neck to reduce blood pressure are called:
 a. vasodilators.
 b. beta blockers.
 c. **alpha blockers.**
 d. ACE inhibitors.

20. Angina pectoris is a coronary artery disease relieved by taking a(n):
 a. arrhythmic.
 b. **vasodilator.**
 c. beta blocker.
 d. calcium channel blocker.

21. Candidiasis is classified as:
 a. cancer.
 b. shingles.
 c. yeast infection.
 d. **fungal infection.**

22. Shingles is the reactivation of which viral infection?
 a. measles
 b. mumps
 c. influenza
 d. **chicken pox**

23. Hyperglycemia is seen primarily in which type of diabetes?
 a. **Type I**
 b. Type II
 c. gestational
 d. Insulin Resistance

24. The primary cause of Type II diabetes is:
 a. polyuria.
 b. polyphagia.
 c. ketoacidosis.
 d. **insulin resistance.**

25. Which adrenergic receptor is responsible for relaxing smooth muscle?
 a. beta-1
 b. alpha-1
 c. **beta-2**
 d. alpha-2

26. Both Alzheimer disease and Parkinsonism:
 a. involve serotonin deficiency.
 b. are curable with currently available drug therapies.
 c. **are progressive in spite of currently available drug therapies.**
 d. contain a defect in the enzyme that transforms tyramine to dopamine.

27. The normal range for glucose levels are:
 a. 50–70 mg
 b. **70–110 mg**
 c. 150–170 mg
 d. 170–200 mg

Chapter 5: Pharmacology

1. The magnesium component of an antacid is most likely to cause:
 a. constipation.
 b. **diarrhea.**

 c. wheezing.
 d. rash.

2. The study of drugs and their actions on living organisms is:
 a. pharmacokinetics.
 b. pharmacodynamics.
 c. pharmaceuticals.
 d. **pharmacology.**

3. The class of drugs that completely shuts off acid production in the stomach is:
 a. H2 blockers.
 b. antacids.
 c. **proton pump inhibitors.**
 d. laxatives.

4. The most common side effect of antibiotics is:
 a. **skin rash.**
 b. phototoxicity.
 c. GI tract upset.
 d. hepatotoxicity.

5. A reference used more in a community pharmacy than in a hospital pharmacy is:
 a. *PDR.*
 b. ***Drug Topics Red Book.***
 c. *Ident-A-Drug.*
 d. *Facts & Comparisons.*

6. Drugs have many actions. The desired action is called:
 a. side effect.
 b. physiological effect.
 c. serendipitous effect.
 d. **therapeutic effect.**

7. There are three phases oral drugs pass through in the body. The phase in which the drug is dissolved so the body can absorb it is called the:
 a. pharmacokinetic phase
 b. pharmacodynamic phase
 c. absorption phase
 d. **pharmaceutic phase**

8. Proper blood clotting is dependent on which vitamin?
 a. vitamin D
 b. **vitamin K**
 c. vitamin B_1
 d. vitamin A

9. Drugs originally prescribed to treat hypertension that are now being given to relax smooth muscle in vascular walls are:
 a. **alpha blockers.**
 b. beta blockers.
 c. thiazide diuretics.
 d. loop diuretics.

10. A reference used to identify a specific tablet or capsule by its color and shape is:
 a. *PDR.*
 b. *Facts & Comparisons.*
 c. ***Ident-A-Drug.***
 d. *Drug Topics Red Book.*

11. The drug of choice to treat patients allergic to sulfa is:
 a. erythromycin.
 b. **nitrofurantoin.**

c. erythromycin.
d. metronidazole.

12. An adverse effect of a drug is considered a/an:
    a. poisoning, harmful or life threatening.
    b. anticipated and desired effect.
    c. nuisance factor.
    d. **undesired effect that requires modification of treatment.**

13. The process of how drugs are handled in the body is called:
    a. pharmacology.
    b. pharmacodynamics.
    c. **pharmacokinetics.**
    d. pharmacotherapeutics.

14. The primary site of metabolic processing is the:
    a. **liver.**
    b. kidney.
    c. small intestine.
    d. large intestine.

15. Patients who are taking tetracycline should avoid:
    a. iron supplements.
    b. vitamin B.
    c. zinc.
    d. **sunshine.**

16. The *Physicians' Desk Reference* (PDR) is updated:
    a. monthly.
    b. quarterly.
    c. weekly.
    d. **annually.**

17. Drugs go through four processes in the body. Which process converts drugs to compounds to be used by the body?
    a. absorption
    b. distribution
    c. **metabolism**
    d. excretion

18. The element from the diet that is used by the body to produce thyroid hormone is:
    a. sodium.
    b. aluminum.
    c. **iodine.**
    d. calcium.

19. A food restriction for patients taking MAOIs is:
    a. apples.
    b. **fermented cheese.**
    c. green leafy vegetables.
    d. beef.

20. A synergistic drug reaction is defined as:
    a. **a reaction when the combined effect of the two drugs is greater than the separate effects of the two drugs.**
    b. a reaction when the combined effect of the two drugs is equal to the sum of the separate effects of the two drugs.
    c. a reaction in which one drug interferes with the other, causing the effects of one of the drugs to be lessened or neutralized.
    d. none of the above.

21. A reference that is known as one of the "bibles" of pharmacy is:
    a. *PDR.*
    b. *Drug Topics Red Book.*

c. *Ident-A-Drug.*
d. *Facts & Comparisons.*

22. Aspirin should be prescribed with caution for patients taking:
    a. statins.
    b. beta blockers.
    c. **anticoagulants.**
    d. alpha blockers.

23. An analgesic that is relatively free of side effects is:
    a. meperidine.
    b. **acetaminophen.**
    c. morphine.
    d. hydrocodone.

24. Non-drug therapy could include such substances as:
    a. herbs
    b. vitamins.
    c. amino acids.
    d. **all of the above.**

25. Which of the phases that a drug passes through in the body is affected by age?
    a. **pharmacokinetic phase**
    b. pharmacodynamic phase
    c. pharmaceutic phase
    d. absorption phase

Chapter 6: Dosage Forms, Delivery Systems, and Routes of Administration

1. Buccal is a route of administration in which the medication is delivered:
   a. vaginally.
   b. by injection.
   c. **inside the cheek.**
   d. rectally under the tongue.

2. The most rapid route of administration for medication is:
   a. PO.
   b. SL.
   c. **IV.**
   d. IM.

3. Liquids that carry the direction "Shake Well" are usually:
   a. elixirs.
   b. syrups.
   c. solutions.
   d. **suspensions.**

4. There are several different routes of administration. The most common is:
   a. **PO.**
   b. SL.
   c. IV.
   d. IM.

5. Solid forms of oral medication have several advantages. One disadvantage is:
   a. longer shelf life.
   b. little or no taste.
   c. **delayed onset of action.**
   d. convenience of self administration.

6. Which of the following dosage forms is NOT considered topical?
   a. gel
   b. cream
   c. **lozenge**
   d. ointment

7. Sources of drugs include:
   a. plant sources.
   b. animal sources.
   c. synthetic sources.
   d. **all of the above.**

8. The agency that establishes guidelines for approval and use of all drugs in the United States is the:
   a. **FDA.**
   b. DEA.
   c. ATF.
   d. DFA.

9. Semi-synthetic drugs are:
   a. naturally occurring chemicals.
   b. completely artificially created.
   c. artificially created natural chemicals.
   d. **composed of both natural and synthetic molecules.**

10. Enteral medications enter the body through the:
    a. **gastrointestinal tract.**
    b. veins.
    c. rectum.
    d. nose.

11. Parenteral medications are used because:
    a. they bypass the stomach.
    b. they deliver the medication quickly.
    c. they are used by patients who are unable to take medication by mouth.
    d. **all of the above.**

12. Preservatives are often added to medications to:
    a. increase their shelf life.
    b. eliminate the possibility of contamination.
    c. decrease the cost if drugs are produced in larger amounts.
    d. **a and b.**

13. Sublingual tablets are better than solid oral medications in relieving angina attacks because:
    a. They have local effects.
    b. They are more readily available than other oral medications.
    c. **They bypass the stomach entering the bloodstream for quicker relief.**
    d. They are smaller than most other types of tablets and can be swallowed more easily.

14. The inert ingredients in a drug include the:
    a. flavoring.
    b. coloring.
    c. preservative.
    d. **all of the above.**

15. Antibiotics have an automatic stop date of:
    a. 5 days.
    b. 7 days.
    c. 10 days.
    d. **14 days.**

16. There are several common uses of drugs. Therapeutic agents are drugs that:
    a. relieve pain.
    b. **maintain health.**
    c. assist in reaching a diagnosis.
    d. alter physiological functioning to treat a disorder.

17. One of the disadvantages of taking a liquid oral medication is:
    a. faster acting.
    b. **shorter shelf life.**
    c. flexibility in dosing.
    d. all of the above.

18. Robotics are mainly used in many institutional settings for:
    a. dispensing.
    b. IV admixture.
    c. inventory control.
    d. **unit-dose repackaging procedures.**

19. The advantage(s) of taking a controlled-release medication is:
    a. it limits the risk of side effects.
    b. it increases patient compliance.
    c. it allows for less frequent dosing.
    d. **all of the above.**

20. A solution containing water and ethanol is considered:
    a. soluble.
    b. **aqueous.**
    c. homogeneous.
    d. hydroalcoholic.

21. An elixir is a solution that is considered a(n):
    a. extract.
    b. aqueous solution.
    c. **water-based solution.**
    d. hydroalcoholic solution.

22. Sublingual tablets are delivered by dissolving:
    a. topically.
    b. transdermally.
    c. **under the tongue.**
    d. inside the cheek.

23. Enteric coated medications have an advantage because they:
    a. are tasteless.
    b. are faster acting.
    c. dissolve in the stomach.
    d. **dissolve in the intestine.**

24. One type of emulsion form that is considered a single phase is:
    a. **gel.**
    b. jelly.
    c. lotion.
    d. ointment.

25. A dosage form used to deliver medication vaginally or rectally is a(n):
    a. lotion.
    b. elixir.
    c. extract.
    d. **suppository.**

Chapter 7: Pharmacy Calculations and Measurement Systems

1. How many grams of drug in is a 500 mL IV bag labeled 5% Dextrose in water?
   a. 5 g
   b. 15 g
   c. 25 g
   d. 50 g

2. How many grams are in 1700 mg?
   a. 17 g
   b. 1.7 g
   c. 1,700,000 g
   d. 0.17 g

3. Calculate the dosage and mL/hr flow rate for the following drug. Propofol 5 mcg/kg/min is ordered for an 80.3 kg patient. The solution strength is 1 g/100 mL D5W.
   a. 5 mL/hr
   b. 10 mL/hr
   c. 40 mL/hr
   d. 2 mL/hr

4. Calculate the flow rate in gtt/min for an IV infusing 100 mL/hour using a 10 gtt/mL set. The resulting flow rate is:
   a. 60 gtt/min
   b. 17 gtt/min
   c. 20 gtt/min
   d. 4 gtt/min

5. Determine the BSA for a child whose weight is 35.9 kg and height is 63.5 cm.
   a. 0.80 m²
   b. 0.85 m²
   c. 1.50 m²
   d. 1.16 m²

6. Convert 75° Celsius to Fahrenheit.
   a. 157° F
   b. 164° F
   c. 167° F
   d. 183° F

7. Convert 33.2 kg to pounds.
   a. 15 lb
   b. 17 lb
   c. 33 lb
   d. 73 lb

8. Convert 45 mL to tablespoon(s).
   a. 2 tbs
   b. 3 tbs
   c. 9 tbs
   d. 12 tbs

9. Convert 35° Fahrenheit to Celsius.
   a. 2° C
   b. 6° C
   c. 4° C
   d. 10° C

10. Calculate the completion time for the following infusion. An IV with a restart time of 9:07 p.m. has an infusion time of 6 hr 27 min.
    a. 3:34 p.m.
    b. 12:37 p.m.
    c. 3:34 a.m.
    d. 2:34 p.m.

11. Convert 90 mL to ounces.
    a. 27 oz
    b. 30 oz
    c. 15 oz
    d. 3 oz

12. Change 5:15 to a percentage.
    a. 3%
    b. 33.3%
    c. 39%
    d. 45%

13. How many mcg are in 65 mg?
    a. 65,000 mcg
    b. 0.065 mcg
    c. 0.65 mcg
    d. 6500 mcg

14. Determine a child's dosage with a BSA of 0.81 m² receiving a drug with a recommended dosage of 40 mg/m².
    a. 30 mg
    b. 35 mg
    c. 32 mg
    d. 33 mg

15. Your stock solution contains 10 mg of active ingredient per 5 mL of carrier vehicle. The physician has ordered a dose of 4 mg. How many mL of stock solution will have to be administered?
    a. 2 mL
    b. 4 mL
    c. 6 mL
    d. 8 mL

16. What is 20% of 60?
    a. 6
    b. 12
    c. 10
    d. 3

17. Your pharmacy has Demerol 100 mg/mL syringes on hand. You receive an order for Demerol 75 mg IM prn pain. How many mL will the nurse give?
    a. 1 mL
    b. 0.2 mL
    c. 0.5 mL
    d. 0.8 mL

18. A suspension of naladixic acid contains 250 mg/5 mL. The syringe contains 15 mL. What is the dose (in milligrams) contained in the syringe?
    a. 750 mg
    b. 500 mg
    c. 725 mg
    d. 250 mg

19. How many 2 tsp doses can a patient take from a bottle containing 3 fl oz?
    a. 10 doses
    b. 5 doses
    c. 9 doses
    d. 12 doses

20. Find the missing term in the ratio. 1:4::x:8
    a. 4
    b. 5
    c. 6
    d. 2

21. Calculate the dosage and mL/hr flow rate for Nipride 3 mcg/kg/min has been ordered for an 87.4 kg patient. The solution has a strength of 50 mg, Nipride in 250 mL D5W.
    a. **79 mL/hr**
    b. 78 mL/hr
    c. 80 mL/hr
    d. 77 mL/hr

22. A 10% solution of 200 mL contains how many grams of drug?
    a. 10 g
    b. 15 g
    c. **20 g**
    d. 2 g

23. An I.V. additive has a dosage available of 30 mEq/20 mL. A dosage of 15 mEq has been ordered. How many mL will you give?
    a. 5 mL
    b. 7 mL
    c. **10 mL**
    d. 15 mL

24. Determine the BSA for an adult whose weight is 175 lb and height is 67 inches.
    a. 1.80 m^2
    b. 1.81 m^2
    c. 1.93 m^2
    d. **1.94 m^2**

25. A critical care patient has orders for a continuous morphine drip. The order is for 25 mg/50 mL to infuse at 8 mg/hr. Calculate the mL/hr flow rate.
    a. 8 mL/hr
    b. **16 mL/hr**
    c. 5 mL/hr
    d. 6 mL/hr

26. Convert 3500 mg to grams
    a. 0.35 g
    b. 35 g
    c. **3.5 g**
    d. 350 g

27. The doctor ordered 0.015 g of Inderal. How many milligrams is the pharmacy technician going to dispense?
    a. 1.5 mg
    b. 0.15 mg
    c. 150 mg
    d. **15 mg**

28. Convert 20° Fahrenheit to Celsius
    a. 7° C
    b. 17° C
    c. **−7° C**
    d. −17° C

29. The pharmacy technician is asked to prepare a 3% ointment of 45 grams. The stock on hand is 10% ointment and 1% ointment. What is the final weight of the 10% ointment?
    a. **10 g**
    b. 100 g
    c. 5 g
    d. 15 g

30. Change the 2:5 to a percentage
    a. 20%
    b. 250%
    c. **40%**
    d. 15%

31. Change the ratio 21:35 into a fraction
    a. 3/4
    b. 1/5
    c. 1/4
    d. **3/5**

32. Convert 120 mL to ounces.
    a. **4 oz**
    b. 24 oz
    c. 12 oz
    d. 15 oz

33. The pharmacy receives an order for a 30 day supply of Lasix 10 mg to be given four times a day. How many tablets must the technician prepare?
    a. 50 tablets
    b. 100 tablets
    c. **120 tablets**
    d. 90 tablets

34. How many milliliters is in 20 liters?
    a. 2000 mL
    b. **20,000 mL**
    c. 200 mL
    d. 200,000 mL

35. An IV of 200 mL of 10% Dextrose was discontinued after only 150 mL had been infused. How many grams of dextrose was delivered?
    a. 5 g
    b. 50 g
    c. 25 g
    d. **15 g**

36. Convert 24 pounds to kilograms
    a. 11.2 kg
    b. **10.9 kg**
    c. 12.4 kg
    d. 52.8 kg

37. Determine the body surface area of a child who weighs 35.9 kg and 63.5 cm in height.
    a. 0.63 m^2
    b. 0.61 m^2
    c. **0.8 m^2**
    d. 0.82 m^2

38. An adult is to receive a drug with a recommend dosage of 10–20 units per m^2. The BSA is 1.93 m^2. What is the recommended range for this patient?
    a. **19–39 units**
    b. 20–38 units
    c. 9–18 units
    d. 18–38 units

39. How much sodium chloride is in 250 mL of D5NS?
    a. 22.5 g
    b. 2.5 g
    c. 2 g
    d. 12.5 g

40. Divide 700 by 1800 and express the answer to the nearest tenth.
    a. 0.38
    b. 0.39
    c. 0.4
    d. 0.3

41. How many micrograms are in 30 milligrams?
    a. 300 mcg
    b. 0.03 mcg
    c. 0.3 mcg
    d. 30,000 mcg

42. A dosage of 0.2 g has been ordered. The strength available is 0.5 g/5 mL. How many milliliters needs to be prepared?
    a. 2 mL
    b. 2.5 mL
    c. 3 mL
    d. 4 mL

43. Convert a child weighing 25.3 kg to pounds.
    a. 55 lb
    b. 50 lb
    c. 54 lb
    d. 56 lb

44. Calculate the BSA of a man weighting 108 kg and whose height is 194 cm.
    a. 5.82 m²
    b. 58.2 m²
    c. 2.41 m²
    d. 24.1 m²

45. The pharmacy receives an order for 1.5 g of Pencillin G to be given by IM. The stock vial contains 500 mg/1 mL. How many milliliters need to be dispensed?
    a. 3 mL
    b. 5 mL
    c. 10 mL
    d. 15 mL

46. Convert the weight of a 125 lb adult to kilograms.
    a. 52.7 kg
    b. 55.4 kg
    c. 56.8 kg
    d. 57.2 kg

47. Calculate the BSA for an adult weighting 165 lb and is 67" in height.
    a. 1.87m²
    b. 1.88m²
    c. 1.89m²
    d. 1.92m²

48. An IV medication of 25 mL is order to infuse in 30 min. The set calibration is 60 gtt/mL. Calculate the gtt/min flow rate.
    a. 15 gtt/min
    b. 20 gtt/min
    c. 30 gtt/min
    d. 50 gtt/min

49. Convert 30 mL to teaspoon(s).
    a. 2 tsp
    b. 4 tsp
    c. 6 tsp
    d. 8 tsp

50. The pharmacy technician is asked to prepare an injection of Thorazine(r) 30mg from a stock vial of 25mg/mL. How many milliliters will the technician draw up?
    a. 0.5 mL
    b. 1.1 mL
    c. 1.2 mL
    d. 1.5 mL

51. How would 8:30 PM be expressed in 24-hour time?
    a. 21:30
    b. 2200
    c. 2130
    d. 22:00

Chapter 8: Sterile Products and Pharmacy Equipment

1. All manipulations inside an LAH should be performed at least ____ inches inside the hood to prevent ____.
    a. 12 inches; smoke
    b. 6 inches; contamination
    c. 10 inches; contamination
    d. 2 inches; breakage from falling on the floor

2. An ampule is composed entirely of glass. Once broken, it:
    a. becomes an open system
    b. remains a closed system
    c. turns into a multiple dose solution
    d. none are correct

3. IV tubing used as a primary set includes which of the following?
    a. macro drop tubing (delivering 10 gtt/min)
    b. micro drip tubing (delivering 60 gtt/min)
    c. all purpose tubing (delivering 100 gtt/min)
    d. both a & b

4. To assure the sterility of a new needle:
    a. wipe the needle with 70% isopropyl to disinfect it
    b. apply additional silicone so the needle self sterilizes upon insertion into a vial
    c. only open the package in a clean room
    d. make sure the package was intact and not damaged

5. IV fluid should hang how many inches higher than the patient's bed?
    a. 12 inches
    b. 24 inches
    c. 36 inches
    d. 49 inches

6. The piggyback is placed ____ the primary IV.
    a. Lower than
    b. higher than
    c. at the same height as
    d. away from

7. Ampules differ from vials in that they:
   a. are closed systems
   b. require the use of a filter needle
   c. can be opened without risk of breakage
   d. do not differ from vials

8. The labeling of an IV admixture should contain all of the following information *except*:
   a. patient name
   b. name and amount of drug(s) added
   c. prescribing physician's name
   d. expiration date

9. Dextrose is the base component of TPN solutions that are most commonly given as a source of carbohydrates. Which of the following statements are true?
   a. Dextrose is available in a concentrated form (50% or more) that is diluted in the final TPN solution to approximately 25%
   b. Dextrose is available as a 5% solution that is commonly used as is in TPN solutions
   c. Dextrose is available as a 70% solution that is commonly given as a separate infusion for calories and energy
   d. all of the above

10. The CADD is an example of what type of pump system?
    a. mechanical system
    b. ambulatory electronic infusion pump system
    c. electronic controlled pressure and chemical release system
    d. none of the above

11. The most common complication of tunneled venous access devices are:
    a. catheter occlusion
    b. infections
    c. dislodgement
    d. venous thrombosis

12. The space between the HEPA filter and the sterile product being prepared is referred to as the:
    a. hot spot
    b. backwash zone
    c. zone of turbulence
    d. critical area

13. Electrolytes are added to TPN solutions to meet metabolic needs and correct deficiencies. Examples of electrolytes include:
    a. potassium chloride
    b. amino acids
    c. vitamin D
    d. lipid emulsions

14. Lipid or fat emulsions are typically administered by all of the following methods *except*:
    a. as a 10% emulsion given through a peripheral line
    b. as a 20% emulsion given through a peripheral line
    c. as part of an IV push
    d. as part of a 3-in-1 solution

15. Preservatives in parenteral products:
    a. kill organisms and eliminate the need for aseptic technique and LAHs
    b. are present in multi-dose vials

c. are harmless and non-toxic in any amount
d. all of the above are correct

16. Items inside an LAH should be placed away from other objects and the walls of the hood to prevent:
    a. zones of turbulence
    b. windows of contamination
    c. dead space
    d. laminar air zones

17. Mixing of 3-in-1 solutions should be performed carefully to prevent the emulsion from "oiling out." It is recommended that this be accomplished by:
    a. preparing the solution in a very cold room
    b. preparing the solution from fresh lipids
    c. using a mixing order of fats, amino acids, and dextrose
    d. using a mixing order of dextrose, fats, and then amino acids

18. After a cytotoxic agent is prepared in the pharmacy, transportation:
    a. should be done immediately
    b. should be done in a way as to minimize breakage
    c. includes making the transporter aware of what they are carrying and what the procedure would be in the event of a spill
    d. both b & c

19. Protective apparel for those preparing cytotoxic or hazardous injections in a BSC includes:
    a. a low permeability, solid front gown with tight fitting elastic cuffs
    b. latex gloves
    c. a self-contained respirator
    d. both a & b

20. Needle sizes are described by two numbers. The ___ corresponds to the diameter of its bore. The ____ measures the shaft.
    a. length; gauge
    b. gauge; length
    c. gauge; tip
    d. depth; length

21. Human touch contamination is the most common source of IV related contamination.
    a. true
    b. false

22. There are two types of area used for compounding in the home care setting. The area that is controlled for microorganisms within designated specifications is called:
    a. sterile compounding area
    b. clean compounding area
    c. bacteria free area
    d. clean room

23. Sterile products should be prepared in a "class 100" environment. In most pharmacies this is accomplished with the use of a:
    a. room air filter
    b. fan cycling air 100 times per hour
    c. laminar Air Flow Hood (LAH)
    d. fume hood

24. In the typical IV setup, an LVP is attached to a primary set, which is then attached to the catheter and inserted into the patient. Drugs administered intermittently are usually given:
    a. **through a Y-site injection port or flashball on the primary set**
    b. by adding them to the LVP solution
    c. through another IV line (not through the one used for the LVP)
    d. through the same site as the primary IV

25. Large volume parenteral solution containers with potent drugs that need to be infused with a high degree of accuracy and precision are usually administered with the aid of a:
    a. roller clamp
    b. **electronic infusion device**
    c. hand clamp
    d. counting device controlled by the nurse

Chapter 9: Preparation of Non-Sterile Products

1. The most commonly compounded formulations are:
   a. ointment
   b. tablets
   c. **solutions**
   d. lotions

2. The most common solvent for oral solutions is:
   a. alcohol
   b. glycerin
   c. syrups
   d. **water**

3. The minimum amount of alcohol required to preserve solutions if no other preservatives are present is:
   a. **15%**
   b. 20%
   c. 25%
   d. 30%

4. Which of the steps listed below is part of the process of preparing an oral suspension from a tablet?
   a. powdering of tablets with a mortar and pestle
   b. wet the powder to make a paste
   c. dilute the wet powder to the desired concentration
   d. **all of the above**

5. Which of the following results in the most wasted product:
   a. extemporaneous
   b. repackaging
   c. **batching**
   d. none of the above

6. The expiration date given to oral solids that are repackaged is:
   a. One year from the date of repackaging
   b. **Six months from the date of repackaging or 25% of the remaining time between the date of repackaging and the expiration date of the oral solid**
   c. Six months from the date of repackaging
   d. 25% of the remaining time between the date of repackaging and the expiration date of the oral solid

7. The organization responsible for providing the guidelines for manufacturers that package medications is the:
   a. Drug Enforcement Agency
   b. Bureau of Manufacturers
   c. The United States Pharmacopeia
   d. **Food and Drug Administration**

8. Scales differ in their range of weight. When weighing 150 mg of medication, the technician should use:
   a. **a class A balance**
   b. a class B balance
   c. a class C balance
   d. either a class A or B balance

9. A graduate is defined as:
   a. a concave container used to mix liquids
   b. **a calibrated measuring container used to mix liquids**
   c. a container used to mix larger products that require high-speed blending
   d. instrument used to stir products such as suspensions

10. The weights of a balance are very sensitive. The technician must use tweezers to prevent:
    a. improper measurement of medication
    b. offsetting the measurement of medication
    c. **altering the exact weight of the metal**
    d. prevent oils from the hands getting onto the metal

11. Of the information listed below, which one is not required to apply on the label of a unit dose item?
    a. name of the drug
    b. dosage strength
    c. expiration date
    d. **patient's name**

12. The definition of levigation is:
    a. **triturating a powder drug with a solvent in which it is insoluble to reduce its particle size**
    b. the fine grinding of a powder
    c. a technique for mixing two powders of unequal size
    d. fully and evenly combining a mixture

13. When a solution at room temperature has absorbed all of the solute it can, it is called a:
    a. supersaturated solution
    b. complete solution
    c. **saturated solution**
    d. soluble solution

14. Of the following capsules, which one would hold the least volume?
    a. size 0
    b. size 1
    c. size 4
    d. **size 5**

15. The method a technician uses to fill a capsule is called the:
    a. slide method
    b. **punch method**
    c. fill method
    d. cake method

16. When combining drugs in a mortar and pestle, the most potent ingredient or the ingredient that occurs in the smallest amount is placed in the mortar:

a. first
b. last
c. part of the medication at the beginning and part at the end
d. in small amounts throughout the process

17. An ingredient dissolved in a solution is known as a:
a. **solute**
b. solvent
c. suspension
d. emulsion

18. In order to _____, a suppository-forming liquid is immediately poured into a mold.
a. prevent contamination
b. mix the ingredients
c. prevent exposure to the air
d. **solidify the suppository**

19. When placing weights on a balance, they should always be placed:
a. **on the right hand side**
b. on the left hand side
c. using a spatula
d. with gloves

20. When measuring small amount of liquid, it is best to use a:
a. cylindrical graduate
b. conical graduate
c. **pipette**
d. medicine dropper

21. The zero point of a balance scale is called:
a. equal point
b. **equilibrium**
c. levigation
d. counter balance

22. A compounding slab is also called a:
a. porcelain slab
b. clean slab
c. sterile slab
d. **ointment slab**

23. When preparing a suspension, an auxiliary label should be applied to the container that states:
a. Take only with food
b. Take on an empty stomach
c. **Shake Well**
d. Take with a large amount of water

24. While pouring a liquid slowly into a graduate, the measurement should be:
a. **observed on eye level**
b. observed by looking down into the graduate
c. reading the level of the liquid from the top of the meniscus
d. all of the above are acceptable

25. The type of mortar and pestle used to mix suspensions or porous liquids is:
a. porcelain
b. **glass**
c. plastic
d. china

Chapter 10: Dispensing Medications

1. The automatic stop date for antibiotics is:
a. one week.
b. **two weeks.**
c. three weeks.
d. determined by the prescribing physician.

2. Which of the following is an illegal activity for a pharmacy technician?
a. obtaining laboratory results
b. **providing counseling for a patient**
c. screening orders for nonformulary/restricted drugs
d. taking medication orders from a medical office

3. Which of the following is NOT required for authorization to release patient information?
a. a hand-written copy
b. a signature
c. **a list of the patient's medications**
d. a reason for release

4. Which of the following may need to be labeled with a federal "transfer warning"?
a. schedule III drugs
b. schedule IV drugs
c. schedule V drugs
d. **All of the above**

Schedule V controlled substances are considered OTC. They are classified as a scheduled drug because they contain a form of:
a. Demerol.
b. morphine.
c. **codeine.**
d. oxycodone.

5. Of the information listed below, which is vital before you can fill a patient's prescription?
a. address
b. full name
c. insurance number or medical record number
d. **all of the above**

6. What is the maximum number of refills for a Schedule II prescription order?
a. six months or five refills
b. as many refills as the physician indicates
c. twice a year
d. **no refills**

7. What should a pharmacist look for when determining the validity of a prescription?
a. an indication not found in the package insert
b. significantly more orders from one prescriber compared to others in the prescriber's area
c. prescription orders written in the names of other people
d. **all of the above**

8. What is the maximum number of refills that you can dispense for a Schedule IV prescription order?
a. none
b. one refill within one month from the date written
c. **five refills within six months from the date written**
d. unlimited refills within one year

9. How many times can a patient transfer among pharmacies a refillable prescription for a Schedule III or IV controlled substance?
   a. **as many times as the prescription is refillable if the pharmacies share an electronic real-time database**
   b. three times between non-related, non-networked pharmacies
   c. as often as the patient and prescriber agree
   d. controlled substances are non-transferable

10. A prescription label must contain all of the following information EXCEPT the:
    a. name and address of the pharmacy.
    b. name of the prescriber.
    c. directions for use with precautions.
    d. **time it was filled.**

11. One way to detect a forged prescription is to check to see if the:
    a. prescription is folded.
    b. prescription was written several days ago.
    c. directions are written with no abbreviations used.
    d. **indications on the description match those of the package insert.**

12. How long of a supply can you give, under the pharmacist's discretion, for an emergency refill of a Schedule II medication?
    a. **72 hours**
    b. 24 hours
    c. one week
    d. none – refills without authorization is illegal

13. You should perform all the following prevention techniques EXCEPT:
    a. knowing the prescriber's DEA number.
    b. **calling the prescriber for verification after dispensing the medication.**
    c. asking for proper identification.
    d. calling the doctor if you believe the patient has forged a prescription.

14. Which of the following must be on the label of an over-the-counter medication container?
    a. manufacturer's name
    b. expiration date
    c. established name of all active ingredients
    d. **all of the above**

15. Investigational drugs are drugs that:
    a. have recently received approval from the FDA for human use.
    b. **have not received approval from the FDA for human use.**
    c. do not require approval from the FDA.
    d. are only available for terminally ill patients.

16. You can assess a customer's ability to learn by evaluating all of the following EXCEPT:
    a. if the patient has a learning impairment.
    b. **if the patient is left-handed or right-handed.**
    c. if the patient has difficulty reading.
    d. the education level of the patient.

17. Which of the following is an accurate description of how the DEA assigns an identity to a prescriber?
    a. The DEA randomly assigns a number.
    b. The first two letters are the prescriber's initials. The numbers are randomly assigned.
    c. **The first letter determines the prescriber's practice. The second letter is the first letter of the prescriber's last name. The seven numbers are determined by adding the first, third, and fifth number. Add the second, fourth, and sixth number and multiply by two. Add the two sums together. The final number should match the last digit of the DEA number.**
    d. The first two letters are the prescriber's initials. The seven numbers are determined by the first six numbers. The last digit should match the last digit of the DEA number.

18. Which of the following patients would benefit from medication bottles that come in different shapes and sizes?
    a. an elderly patient
    b. a hearing-impaired patient
    c. **a visually-impaired patient**
    d. a patient with a different cultural background

Chapter 11: Inventory Management and Handling and Storage of Medications

1. Prescriptions come into the pharmacy in a variety of ways. The most common is by:
   a. **walk-ins.**
   b. physician's phone in.
   c. fax.
   d. none of the above.

2. Which of the following medications must have a federal "transfer warning" label unless they are dispensed and administered by a healthcare facility?
   a. Schedule II drugs
   b. Schedule III drugs
   c. Schedule IV drugs
   d. **all of the above**

3. How often must a pharmacy perform a controlled substance inventory?
   a. yearly
   b. **every two years**
   c. every three years
   d. monthly

4. Which medication dispensing unit is excellent for bulk storage, but not for unit-dose storage?
   a. cassette systems
   b. medication carts
   c. **stationary wall units**
   d. floor stock

5. A technicians' duty with regard to over-the-counter drugs typically include(s):
   a. stocking.
   b. taking inventory.
   c. removing expired drugs from the shelves.
   d. **all of the above.**

6. The most common reason drugs are returned to the manufacturer is because:
   a. they are recalled.
   b. they are expired.
   c. the wrong product is ordered.
   d. they are mislabeled.

7. Which of the following methods of maintaining a formulary is the most convenient and yields the most current product information in a purchasing and inventory system?
   a. computerized formulary
   b. formulary log book
   c. want book
   d. log book

8. When documenting the receipt of pharmaceuticals for which the purchase order or manufacturer's invoice cannot be located, which of the following information should be recorded?
   a. product name and amount
   b. product name, strength, and amount
   c. date of receipt, name of receiver, product name, strength, dosage form, and amount
   d. name of wholesaler, product name, strength, dosage form, and amount

9. When controlled substances are stored in a pharmacy, where may they be kept?
   a. in a locked cabinet
   b. dispersed throughout the inventory of non-controlled drugs
   c. in a separate locked room
   d. either a or b

10. Formularies are typically updated every:
    a. 4–6 months.
    b. 12–18 months.
    c. 18–24 months.
    d. 3–4 years.

11. The type of inventory method used for controlled substances is called:
    a. stock rotation inventory.
    b. controlled inventory.
    c. perpetual inventory.
    d. closed inventory.

12. Which type of drugs can be returned to the manufacturer for credit?
    a. investigational
    b. controlled substances
    c. chemicals
    d. bulk

13. When the quantity of a pharmaceutical product in stock reaches a predetermined point, it is called a(n):
    a. stock level.
    b. par level.
    c. maximum level.
    d. ideal level.

14. The most important consideration in processing a manufacturer's recall notice is:
    a. timely response in checking the inventory.
    b. timely response in removing affected products from the inventory.

c. receiving proper credit from the manufacturer.
d. both a and b.

15. Which of the following statements about prescription labeling is false?
    a. Some prescriptions require labeling beyond what will fit on the label itself.
    b. Auxiliary labels are often used to clarify or elaborate on directions for use.
    c. If the patient is in a hurry, it is acceptable to dispense the prescription without an affixed label as long as the pharmacist talks to the patient about how to use the medication and he/she understands the directions.
    d. Most states have specific requirements about what information must be include in prescription labeling.

16. Temperature is very important for the storage of medication. Room temperature is considered to be:
    a. 15° to 30°C or 59° to 86°F.
    b. 2° to 8°C or 36° to 46°F.
    c. 30° to 40°C or 86° to 104°F.
    d. Above 40°C or 104°F.

17. Which of the following best incorporates all recommended components of label directions for outpatient use?
    a. Take one tablet three times daily.
    b. Take one tablet by mouth three times daily for 10 days for infection.
    c. Take one tablet by mouth three times daily for 10 days.
    d. Take one tablet three times daily for pain.

18. A situation that might require adjustment of the pharmacy's inventory level on a short-term basis is:
    a. an increased need for seasonal products, such as asthma medication.
    b. a particular patient requiring high doses of a pain medication.
    c. an extended period of high use of a particular product by multiple patients.
    d. a and b.

19. The NDC number is assigned by the manufacturer for each drug it produces. What do the individual digits in the NDC number mean?
    a. The first five digits indicate the manufacturer, the next four indicate the medication, its strength, and dosage form, and the last two digits indicate the package size.
    b. The first five digits indicate the medication, its strength, and dosage form, the next four indicate the package size, and the last two indicate the manufacturer.
    c. The first five digits indicate the manufacturer, the next four indicate the package size, and the last two indicate the medication, its strength, and dosage form.
    d. The first five digits indicate the medication, its strength, and dosage form, the next four indicate the manufacturer, and the last two indicate the package size.

20. A package insert is always dispensed to the patient for which type of medication?
    a. high blood pressure
    b. estrogens
    c. diabetic
    d. psychotropic

21. Newly acquired products will generally have a longer shelf life and should be placed behind packages that will expire before them. This procedure is called:
    a. overstocking.
    b. inventory rotation.
    c. **stock rotation.**
    d. perpetual inventory process.

22. The Occupational Safety and Health Administration (OSHA) requires pharmacies to have this on hand for each hazardous chemical they use:
    a. **Material Safety Data Sheets**
    b. United States Pharmacopoeia Drug Information
    c. Pharmacy Law Digest
    d. Facts and Comparisons

23. Inventory control may include:
    a. maintaining minimum and maximum reorder points.
    b. returning outdated stock.
    c. recording the receipt of controlled substances.
    d. **all of the above.**

24. The form used to order Schedule II drugs from a wholesaler or supplier is called:
    a. DEA form 203.
    b. **DEA form 222.**
    c. DEA form 124.
    d. DEA form 320.

25. The DEA form consists of how many parts?
    a. Two parts; the pharmacy keeps one part and returns the second one to the wholesaler.
    b. Four parts; the pharmacy keeps one part, returns the second one to the wholesaler, and the remaining two go to the DEA.
    c. One part, which stays with the pharmacy as the wholesaler already has a duplicate copy.
    d. **Three parts; the pharmacy keeps one part, two are returned to the wholesaler with one copy being sent to DEA.**

Chapter 12: Administrative Duties and Technology

1. Licensing and general professional oversight of pharmacists and pharmacies is carried out by:
    a. College of Pharmacy
    b. The American Pharmaceutical Society
    c. The United States Pharmacopoeia Convention
    d. **State pharmacy boards**

2. The purpose of the clinical pharmacy is to:
    a. dispense medications
    b. **provide information about medication**
    c. compound medication
    d. report adverse reaction or interactions of medication

3. At present, no federal requirements and few state requirements exist for the training and licensing of pharmacy technicians.
    a. **true**
    b. false

4. A person who assists professionals in carrying out their duties is called a
    a. druggist
    b. toxicologist

c. paraprofessional
    d. none of the above

5. A technician carries out many of the same duties as a pharmacist and depending on the facility can dispense medication without the supervision of a pharmacist.
    a. true
    b. **false**

6. Of the automated systems listed, which is the most commonly used to manage controlled substances levels?
    a. Pyxis machine
    b. Baker Cell System
    c. Bar coding
    d. **both a and c**

7. A set of standards used to prepare medications that lower the possibility of contamination is:
    a. **universal precautions**
    b. aseptic technique
    c. guidelines for handwashing
    d. guidelines for hood cleaning

8. In a hospital, the overall responsibility for the materials management of pharmaceuticals lies with the:
    a. Chairman of the Pharmacy and Therapeutics Committee
    b. Hospital Board of Directors
    c. **Director of Pharmacy Services**
    d. Materials Manager

9. When a filling label seems to indicate an error, which of the following would be an appropriate initial action for the technician?
    a. **alert the pharmacist that an error has been made**
    b. check the label against the original order to determine if an error was made
    c. call the physician to clarify the order
    d. call the nursing unit (institutional setting) or notify the patient (outpatient setting) that an error was made on the prescription order

10. Besides choosing the correct drug entity, which of the following decisions must be made at the time an IV drug is being chosen during a computerized order entry process in the hospital?
    a. the correct dosage for the amount being prepared
    b. the correct dosage form for the route of administration
    c. the correct dilute solution
    d. **all of the above**

11. An example of the automation machines used to prepare hyperalimentation solutions is/are:
    a. Robot-Rx
    b. **MicroMix and AutoMix**
    c. SureMed
    d. none of the above

12. Which of the following statements regarding quality is *false*?
    a. quality control is a process of checks and balances
    b. quality may be defined by what customers perceive
    c. **because quality is something that cannot be directly measured, it is more important to focus on the quantity of products made**
    d. quality is determined by the cleanliness of the pharmacy

13. Which of the following is *not* true of hospital pharmacy dispensing automation?
    a. both centralized and decentralized automation make dispensing more efficient
    b. decentralized automation is superior to centralized automation
    c. some institutions combine both centralized and decentralized automation to incorporate advantages of both systems
    d. dispensing automation may be centralized in the pharmacy or decentralized at the point of care

14. Any suspicious prescription should be brought to the attention of the pharmacist because it may be a forgery.
    a. true
    b. false

15. Which of the following statements regarding pharmacy directors is *false*?
    a. pharmacy directors often report to one of the hospital's administrators
    b. pharmacy directors are at the top of the pharmacy department's personnel
    c. pharmacy directors are responsible for the activity within the pharmacy
    d. pharmacy directors can operate all activities independent of other departments or managers

16. A pharmacy technician is preparing a 1-week supply of total parenteral nutrition for a patient at home using an automated compounding device. Investigational L-glutamine is being added at the end of the mixing process. Which risk level of compounding describes this situation?
    a. Immediate-use
    b. Low-risk
    c. Medium-risk
    d. High-risk

17. A flexible spending account requires:
    a. the employee to pay a co-pay for their provider services
    b. the employer to set aside a portion of an employees earning for qualified expenses
    c. the physician to pay an annual fee to participate in the insurance plan
    d. the patient to pay out-of-pocket for services and then submits a receipt to the insurance plan for reimbursement

18. Which of the following statements about CQI is/are *false*?
    a. CQI focuses on people problems
    b. CQI allows decisions to be made on the basis of objective data alone
    c. CQI is a scientific/systematic approach to quality
    d. a & b

19. What are the two major mechanisms for third-party pharmacy reimbursement?
    a. POS and fee-for-service
    b. capitation and POS
    c. copayments and deductibles
    d. fee-for-service and capitation

20. Which of the following *is not* a copayment arrangement designated by third parties?
    a. fee-for-service
    b. flat rate

    c. variable rate
    d. straight percentage

21. Communication skills and customer service are the most important qualifications of a pharmacy technician. Which duty is *not* a responsibility of a technician?
    a. handle demanding patients appropriately
    b. counseling patients on their medication
    c. computer order entry
    d. prescription filling and labeling

22. Access to the pharmacy computer system is controlled by:
    a. finger print touch screen
    b. signature of the pharmacy personnel
    c. user name and password
    d. combination of finger print and signature

23. Current computer technology used in health care today is:
    a. bar coding
    b. touch screens
    c. automated dispensing systems
    d. all of the above

24. Information needed on the patient's medication profile includes all the following *except:*
    a. whether the patient is married or single
    b. dosage strength and form
    c. insurance provider
    d. duration time of medication

25. Which of the following statements is a disadvantage of the robotic cart fill system?
    a. the use of bar coding provides accuracy in identify the patient
    b. good inventory control
    c. special packaging and equipment for the system
    d. removal of expired drugs before they are dispensed

Chapter 13: Business Management

1. There are four main associations concerned with pharmacy practice. Which one listed is *not* a member?
    a. ASHP
    b. APhA
    c. JACHO
    d. AAPT

2. What job responsibility for a technician is found in an inpatient setting, but not in a community setting?
    a. insurance billing technician
    b. IV technician
    c. stock inventory technician
    d. technician recruiter

3. Health care institutions are usually organized into several levels of management. Which position is not at the top of the institution?
    a. department managers
    b. CEO
    c. COO
    d. CFO

4. Policy and procedures manuals exist for which of the following reason(s)?
    a. to serve as a legal document
    b. to prevent error caused by verbal communication

c. to train new employees
d. **all of the above**

5. The definition of a *policy* is:
   a. a way of accomplishing something or acting
   b. **a definite course or method of action selected from among alternatives; a high-level, overall plan**
   c. a series of steps followed in a regular definite order
   d. a traditional or established way of doing things.

6. The Clinical Section of the policy and procedure manual contains those activities involved in patient-related monitoring activities of a clinical nature. Which activity listed is *not* part of this section?
   a. drug ordering
   b. unit-dose drug distribution
   c. **drug information services**
   d. formulary operation

7. A not-for-profit, nongovernmental corporation whose responsibility is to regulate hospital settings is:
   a. **JCAHO**
   b. OSHA
   c. ASHP
   d. NABP

8. The definition of *procedure* is:
   a. a high-level, overall plan embracing the general goals
   b. **a traditional or established way of doing things**
   c. a definite course or method of action
   d. none of the above

9. Regulations affecting pharmacy practice encompass:
   a. CSA regulations
   b. JCAHO standards
   c. federal and state rules
   d. **all of the above**

10. The Administrative section of a policy and procedure manual contain all the following information *except:*
    a. department's hours of operation
    b. inventory control
    c. **drug therapy monitoring**
    d. annual reports

11. Policy and procedure manuals have a standard format. The first item in the manual is:
    a. **title**
    b. table of contents
    c. objectives
    d. goals

12. The liaison between the medical staff and the department of pharmacy services is:
    a. JCAHO
    b. **The pharmacy and Therapeutics Committee**
    c. Medicare
    d. hospital Board of Pharmacy

13. Pharmacy technicians perform essential tasks that do not require:
    a. computer entry training
    b. compounding techniques
    c. label preparation
    d. **the pharmacist's skill or expertise**

14. Pharmacy technicians may use the following designation after their name after passing the Pharmacy Technician National Certification exam:
    a. APhT
    b. **CPhT**
    c. RTech
    d. CPT

15. The members of the Pharmacy & Therapeutic committee review and update the manual every:
    a. year
    b. two years
    c. **5 years**
    d. 18 months

16. The State Boards of Pharmacy have the responsibility of:
    a. dealing with complaints
    b. licensure and registration of pharmacy staff
    c. poison schedules
    d. **all of the above**

17. Which of the following is *not* true regarding policy and procedure manuals?
    a. **any change in the manual requires the approval of the CEO**
    b. they provide job descriptions for new employees
    c. they guarantee accuracy in routine operational activities
    d. they prevent waste of time by providing direction in repetitive tasks

18. The OBRA '90 requires community pharmacists offer:
    a. free samples if the patient cannot afford the medication
    b. **counseling to Medicaid patients regarding their medication**
    c. ordering of all medications
    d. inventory control

19. One of the most positive responses to a dissatisfied a customer is:
    a. listening intently
    b. making eye contact
    c. restating what the customer has to say
    d. **all of the above**

20. If the technician is unable to resolve the customer's problem, he/she should:
    a. **inform the pharmacist**
    b. ask another technician for help
    c. ask to speak to another family member of the customer
    d. ask the customer to leave

Chapter 14: Professionalism and Personnel Management

1. Which of the following statements about quality control is *false*?
   a. Quality control is necessary for IV products because of morbidity and mortality.
   b. **Written policies and procedures are not necessary if a quality control format is in place.**
   c. Quality control builds checks and balances.
   d. All of the above

2. Which of the following statements regarding quality improvement is *false*?
   a. It is an important part of preparation for a JCAHO survey.
   b. It concentrates on problems within the system.
   c. The pharmacy director is totally responsible for quality improvement.
   d. All of the above

3. Laws governing pharmacists, technicians, and other pharmacy personnel are set by
   a. individual state laws
   b. the NABP
   c. the pharmacy itself
   d. professional organizations

4. The organization that certifies pharmacy technicians is
   a. ASHP
   b. NABP
   c. PTCB
   d. APhA

5. Memos can be substituted for policy and procedure updates.
   a. True
   b. False

6. Technicians should familiarize themselves with the administrative and technical aspects of the policy and procedure manual.
   a. True
   b. False

7. The primary goal of pharmacy personnel is communication not only with customers but also with other professionals. Which form of communication is judged by others in the first 30 seconds of meeting?
   a. listening skills
   b. appearance
   c. phone skills
   d. body language

8. Most pharmacies that hire technicians require the same basic skills. Which skill listed is *not* the responsibility of a technician?
   a. troubleshooting third-party prescription claim questions
   b. handling ongoing pharmacy telephone calls
   c. counseling patients on OTC medications
   d. taking in refill prescriptions

9. Many states have laws that differ from federal laws. Pharmacy personnel need to remember
   a. always follow the state law
   b. always follow the strictest law
   c. always follow the federal law
   d. depends on the situation

10. Technicians are monitored in their job performance competency through regularly scheduled performance reviews.
    a. True
    b. False

11. Which system allows for a closer relationship between the pharmacist and medical team, including the patient?
    a. centralized system
    b. decentralized system

c. floor stock system
d. individual prescription orders

12. Although statutes, regulations and standards of practice vary from state to state, under all circumstances, the technician is expected to
    a. work under the supervision of the pharmacist
    b. follow FDA guidelines regarding drug storage
    c. counsel patients on OTC medications
    d. review patient profiles for interactions

13. Technicians have several methods for performance feedback after an evaluation. The most effective method is
    a. faxing your concerns to your supervisor
    b. by preparing a memo
    c. airing your concerns at the time of the evaluation
    d. leaving your concerns on a voice message

14. The most common routine method of communication in the hospital between the pharmacy and the physician is a
    a. prescription
    b. medical order
    c. fax
    d. telephone

15. The State Board of Pharmacy requires that all medication leaving the pharmacy must
    a. be packaged in a proper container
    b. be checked by a pharmacist
    c. be initialed by a technician
    d. all of the above

16. All pharmacy employees are required to be interviewed not only by the pharmacy department by also with
    a. human resources
    b. security
    c. administration
    d. housekeeping

17. Technician training in the pharmacy is usually performed by
    a. the pharmacy manager
    b. outside training coordinator
    c. technician supervisor
    d. none of the above

18. The Policy and Procedure Manual contains information pertaining to
    a. disciplinary actions
    b. performance evaluations
    c. step-by-step directions on how to perform various tasks
    d. all of the above

19. Performance evaluations are usually conducted
    a. monthly
    b. yearly on the technician's starting date
    c. twice a year
    d. bimonthly

Chapter 15: Infection Control and Hazardous Materials

1. The first line of defense in infection control is:
   a. clean apparel
   b. handwashing

c. private rooms for all patients

d. none of the above

2. Hazardous drugs are drugs involved in treating cancer. The term(s) used to describe these drugs is:

a. **chemotherapeutic**

b. statins

c. biguanides

d. aminoglycosides

3. The definition of *nosocomial infection* is:

a. an infection caused by an organism that requires a host for nourishment

b. an infection caused by exposure to a parasite

c. **an infection acquired while hospitalized**

d. an infection acquired by a mosquito bite

4. The type of Laminar Air Hood (LAH) used to prepare cancer medication is:

a. horizontal

b. open

c. **vertical**

d. any of these types of hoods are acceptable

5. When handling antineoplastic medications, the technician usually wears how many pairs of gloves?

a. don't need to wear gloves if the technician is cautious

b. one pair for all drugs

c. don't need to wear gloves if the cuff of the protective gown is long

d. **two pair**

6. Contact with chemotherapy medications can cause:

a. dizziness

b. nausea

c. skin rash

d. **all of the above**

7. When cleaning a laminar airflow hood, the technician must use:

a. **70% isopropyl alcohol**

b. soap and water

c. hot water only

d. any of the above

8. When disposing of sharps, the technician should always clip the needle before placing in the disposal.

a. true

b. **false**

9. ASHP recommends that personnel wash their hands for how long before compounding?

a. **30 seconds**

b. 15 seconds

c. 60 seconds

d. 45 seconds

10. Sterile products should be prepared in a:

a. Class 50 environment

b. Class 75 environment

c. **Class 100 environment**

d. Class 200 environment

11. If skin or eye contact to a hazardous drug occurs, the technician should following these steps:

a. rinse the eye immediately with an eyewash fountain and contact a supervisor

b. establish first aid and document the injury

c. obtain medical attention and document the injury

d. **rinse the eye immediately with an eyewash fountain, obtain medical attention and document the injury**

12. When disposing of hazardous materials, the technician should:

a. dispose the material when container is full

b. **dispose the material separately from other trash**

c. dispose the material with other trash

d. any of the above is appropriate

13. Which of the following is *not* a form of infection transmission in healthcare settings?

a. airborne transmission

b. **otic transmission**

c. droplet transmission

d. contact transmission

14. The difference between bactericidal and bacteriostatic agents is:

a. bactericidal agents prevent the growth of bacteria

b. bacteriostatic agents kill bacteria

c. **bactericidal agents kill bacteria**

d. bactericidal agents are chemical agents produced by organisms used to treat infection

15. In a hospital pharmacy setting, the process most at risk for contamination is:

a. handling drugs

b. liquid preparation

c. compounding

d. **IV preparation**

16. Prior to compounding preparation, the technician needs to clean countertops and equipment with:

a. **alcohol**

b. water

c. warm soap and water

d. any of the above

17. Laminar flow hoods should be cleaned:

a. once a day

b. **at least 30 minutes before using**

c. at least 60 minutes before using

d. twice a day

18. Hands should always be washed or sanitized when:

a. before working in an air flow hood

b. entering the IV room

c. before prepare a compounding medication

d. **all of the above**

19. Which of the skills listed is the *most* important aspect of preparing sterile products?

a. **aseptic technique**

b. using 70% isopropyl alcohol to wipe down the hood

c. discarding of used needles

d. cleaning the surface with soap and water

20. According to USP 797 regulations, what *should not* be worn during compounding preparation?

a. hair ties

b. gloves

c. **artificial nails**

d. all of the above

Chapter 16: Facility Management

1. What duties should a pharmacy technician perform in anticipation of the day in the pharmacy?
   a. make sure the IV clean room is stocked
   b. turn on equipment that will be used throughout the day
   c. turn on Laminar air flow hoods
   d. all of the above

2. The applied science concerned with designing and arranging the equipment personnel use so they can work efficiently and safely is called:
   a. JCAHO compliance
   b. ergonomics
   c. OSHA compliance
   d. Economics

3. How many exits must be designated as fire exits in a pharmacy?
   a. one
   b. three
   c. two
   d. four

4. What class of first extinguisher is used for flammable agents?
   a. Class A
   b. Class B
   c. Class C
   d. Class D

5. Which organization is responsible for making sure pharmacies follow safety guidelines?
   a. OSHA
   b. JCAHO
   c. FDA
   d. DEA

6. A security system that protects pharmacy personnel as well as customers is:
   a. cameras
   b. a common password for only pharmacy personnel
   c. protective glass for pharmacy personnel
   d. all of the above

7. The pharmacy personnel responsible for calibrating and maintaining pharmacy equipment is the:
   a. pharmacy manager
   b. pharmacist in charge
   c. pharmacy technician
   d. building maintenance

8. Pharmacy equipment should have an expiration date of:
   a. six months
   b. one year
   c. two years
   d. three years

9. The *main* purpose of pharmacy equipment is:
   a. accuracy
   b. making the work easier
   c. speed
   d. less cleanup

10. When calibrating the accuracy of a balance, the weights should always be placed on which side of the balance?
    a. left
    b. either
    c. right
    d. combination

11. If a pharmacy technician is unsure about the calibration of a balance, he or she should:
    a. recheck the calibration
    b. consult another technician
    c. consult a pharmacist
    d. any of the above

12. When prepare a compounding medication, a pharmacy technician should clean all equipment with:
    a. warm water
    b. alcohol
    c. soap and water
    d. hot water

13. One of the responsibilities of a hospital technician is the stocking of a crash cart. How does a technician determine whether the cart needs to be restocked?
    a. the pharmacist informs the technician
    b. the nurse informs the technician
    c. the security lock is broken
    d. the technician checks for missing medications daily

14. The red portion of the diamond-shaped warning label on a fire extinguisher signifies:
    a. flammability
    b. health hazards
    c. instability
    d. special hazards

15. The blue portion of the diamond-shaped warning label on a fire extinguisher signifies:
    a. flammability
    b. health hazards
    c. instability
    d. special hazards

16. When using the computer to protect against possible abusers or to record a pharmacy personnel's activities, each authorized person is issued a:
    a. key to turn the computer on
    b. user ID that includes their first initial and last name
    c. password
    d. number

17. Every computer system has a database of information. These files must be:
    a. kept separate
    b. backed up daily
    c. kept in alphabetical order
    d. kept in an operation manual

18. Some drugs must be stored at a constant temperature. If refrigerated, the temperature should be recorded daily and logged generally between:
    a. 22–29°F
    b. 27–32°F

c. 32–38°F
d. 36–46°F

19. A logbook is one way to document routine equipment requirements.
   a. true
   b. false

20. The Americans with Disabilities Act requirements pharmacies to accommodate the disabled by:
   a. providing wheelchair ramps
   b. providing accessible aisles for travel
   c. parking accommodations
   d. all of the above

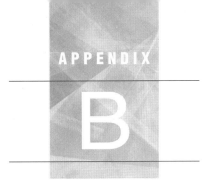

APPENDIX

B

Practice Exam

1. The Occupational and Safety Act was passed to assure:
   a. every working man and woman in the nation has safe and healthful working conditions.
   b. child safety caps are used on all medications in homes where children preside.
   c. pharmacies completed purchase orders according to their state regulations.
   d. customers information is not disclosed to advertising companies.

2. A not-for-profit, nongovernmental corporation whose member organizations are the American College of Physicians, the American College of Surgeons, the American Hospital Association and the American Medical Association
   a. JCAHO
   b. OSHA
   c. HCS
   d. none of the above

3. The brand name for fluticasone is:
   a. Nasonex
   b. Advair
   c. Flovent
   d. Combivent
   e. Nascort AQ

4. All manipulations inside a LAH should be performed at least ___ inches inside the hood to prevent ___.
   a. 12 inches; smoke
   b. 6 inches; backwash
   c. 10 inches; contamination
   d. 2 inches; breakage from falling on the floor

5. Which drug listed below is considered both an immuno-suppressant and an antineoplastic?
   a. Cytoxan
   b. Methotrexate
   c. Azathiprine
   d. Colchicine

6. The brand name for budesonide is:
   a. Pulmicort
   b. Advair
   c. Flovent
   d. Combivent
   e. Nascort AQ

7. In most hospitals, the Pharmacy and Therapeutics Committee (P&T) serves as the:
   a. liaison between the medical staff and the department of pharmacy services.
   b. accreditation body for the pharmacy.
   c. compliant department for the pharmacy staff.
   d. committee that schedules pharmacy vacation days.

8. Policy and procedures manuals exist for the following reasons:
   a. to train new employees or retrain existing employees
   b. to prevent errors that occur due to verbal communication
   c. to serve as legal document in the event of a lawsuit
   d. all of the above

9. The generic name for Combivent is:
   a. fluticasone
   b. triamcinolone
   c. albuterol/ipratropium
   d. fluticasone/salmeterol

10. How many grams are in 1700 mg?
    a. 17 g
    b. 1,700,000 g
    c. 0.17 g
    d. 1.7 g

11. The most common error made in the repackaging process is:
    a. labeling
    b. outdates
    c. recalls
    d. all of the above

12. The brand name for mometasone is:
    a. Tilade
    b. Nasonex
    c. Axmacort
    d. Deltasone
    e. Claritin

13. Calculate the dosage, and mL/hr flow rate for the following drug. Propofol 5 mcg/kg/min is ordered for an 80.3 kg patient. The solution strength is 1 g/100 mL D5W.
    a. 10 mL/hr
    b. 40 mL/hr
    c. 2 mL/hr
    d. none of the above

14. Calculate the infusion time for the following IV medication. A 10 mL volume to infuse at 40 gtt/min using a microdrip. Infusion time is:
    a. 60 gtt/min
    b. 15 gtt/min
    c. 20 gtt/min
    d. 120 gtt/min

15. The brand name for prednisone is:
    a. Tilade
    b. Azmacort

191

c. Claritin
d. Deltasone
e. Nasonex

16. Needle sizes are described by two numbers. The ___ corresponds to the diameter of its bore. The ___ measures the shaft.
   a. length; gauge
   b. gauge; length
   c. neither is correct

17. Ampules are composed entirely of glass and **once broken** it:
   a. remains a closed system
   b. becomes an open system
   c. neither is correct

18. What drug listed below is classified as an antihistamine?
   a. amitryptyline
   b. naproxen
   c. loratadine
   d. sumatriptan

19. A pharmacy technician is asked to prepare a 0.5 mg dosage from a stock strength of 200 mcg/mL. How many milliliters must the technician prepare?
   a. 2 mL
   b. 2.5 mL
   c. 3 mL
   d. 3.5 mL

20. A ___ is a definite course or method of action selected from among alternatives; a high-level, overall plan embracing the general goals and acceptable procedures.
   a. policy
   b. procedure
   c. memo
   d. lesson

21. Fluticasone, triamcinolone and budesonide are classified as:
   a. anticholinergic
   b. leukotriene inhibitors
   c. anti-inflammatory
   d. antiallergic agents

22. Controlled substances are required by federal law to have appropriate safeguards with their use. Which of the following is *not* an issue?
   a. inventory requirements
   b. dispensing records and reports
   c. administration of records and reports
   d. patient consent

23. The disease that occurs when bacteria invades the bone is:
   a. septic arthritis
   b. cellulitis
   c. osteomyelitis
   d. none of the above

24. The brand name for rosiglitazone is:
   a. Orinase
   b. Starlix
   c. Actos
   d. Avandia

25. Determine the BSA for a child whose weight is 35.9 kg and height is 63.5 cm.
   a. 0.80 m^2
   b. 0.85 m^2
   c. 1.50 m^2
   d. 1.16 m^2

26. Determine the BSA for an adult whose weight is 175 lb and height is 67 inches.
   a. 1.94 m^2
   b. 1.93 m^2
   c. 1.80 m^2
   d. 1.81 m^2

27. The generic name for Starlix is:
   a. rosiglitazone
   b. nateglinide
   c. pioglitazone
   d. glimepride

28. Determine the child's dosage for the following drug. A child with a BSA of 0.81 m^2 is to receive a drug with a recommended dosage of 40 mg/m^2.
   a. 27 mg
   b. 30 mg
   c. 32 mg
   d. 40 mg

29. An IV additive has dosage available of 30 mEq per 20 mL. A dosage of 15 mEq has been ordered. How many mL will you give?
   a. 10 mL
   b. 30 mL
   c. 45 mL
   d. 52 mL

30. The brand name for repaglinide is:
   a. Glucophage
   b. Tolinase
   c. Glucotrol
   d. Prandin

31. NSAIDS have three actions called the 3 A's. What action listed below *is not* associated with these actions.
   a. anti-inflammatory
   b. antiemetic
   c. analgesia
   d. antipyretic

32. IV tubing used as a primary set includes which of the following?
   a. macro drip tubing (delivering 10 gtt/min)
   b. micro drip tubing (delivering 60 gtt/min)
   c. all purpose tubing (delivering 100 gtt/min)
   d. both a & b

33. Avandia and Actos are considered to be in which class of diabetic drugs?
   a. Glitazones
   b. Biguanides
   c. Meglitinides
   d. Alpha glucosidase inhibitors

34. Ampules differ from vials in that they:
   a. are closed systems
   b. require the use of a filter needle

c. can be opened without risk of breakage

d. ampules do not differ from vials

35. To assure sterility of a new needle:
    a. the user should make sure the package was intact and not damaged
    b. wipe the needle with 70% isopropyl to disinfect it
    c. apply additional silicone so the needle self sterilizes upon insertion into a vial
    d. ampules do not differ from vials

36. The generic name for Benadryl is:
    a. benzonatate
    b. metclopramide
    c. propranolol
    d. diphenhydramine

37. The most common source of IV related contamination:
    a. human touch
    b. recalls
    c. outdates
    d. wrong drug in the wrong solution

38. IV fluid hang on an IV pole approximately ___ inches higher than the patient's bed.
    a. 12 inches
    b. 24 inches
    c. 36 inches
    d. 49 inches

39. What is the classification of codeine?
    a. beta-blocker
    b. antitussive
    c. tricyclic antidepressant
    d. antihistamine

40. Convert 75 degrees Celsius to Fahrenheit.
    a. 167° F
    b. 157° F
    c. 164° F
    d. 183° F

41. The piggyback is placed ___ than the primary IV.
    a. higher
    b. lower
    c. same height
    d. doesn't make a difference if higher or lower

42. Which of the following drugs in an antihistamine?
    a. Propranolol
    b. Codeine
    c. Sumatriptan
    d. Promethazine

43. Convert 99.2 kilograms to pounds.
    a. 45 lb
    b. 218 lb
    c. 198 lb
    d. 163 lb

44. Convert 33.2 kilograms to pounds.
    a. 15 lb
    b. 17 lb
    c. 73 lb
    d. 75 lb

45. The generic name for Xylocaine is:
    a. Bupivicaine
    b. Lidocaine

c. Benzocaine

d. Lidocaine-prilocaine

46. A ___ prepares medications in a single unit package.
    a. unit-dose drug distribution
    b. single-dose drug distribution
    c. both a & b
    d. neither a nor b

47. There are two types of rooms used for compounding in the home care setting. The ___ is the whole room environment controlled for microorganisms within designated specifications.
    a. clean room
    b. sterile compounding area
    c. clean compounding area
    d. storage room

48. The brand name for Procaine is:
    a. EMLA
    b. Xylocaine
    c. Americaine
    d. Novocain

49. The brand name for rizatriptan is:
    a. Maxalt
    b. Serzone
    c. Orinase
    d. Nascort AQ

50. The *most* common adverse effect of Penicillin:
    a. irritation to the veins
    b. skin rash
    c. blurred vision
    d. n/v

51. The brand name for naproxen is:
    a. Afrin
    b. Elavil
    c. Claritin
    d. Naprosyn

52. Convert 12 tsp to milliliters.
    a. 150 mL
    b. 30 mL
    c. 60 mL
    d. 90 mL

53. Convert 45 mL to tablespoons.
    a. 3 Tbsp
    b. 15 Tbsp
    c. 9 Tbsp
    d. 12 Tbsp

54. The generic name for Claritin is:
    a. divalproex
    b. loratadine
    c. oxymetazoline
    d. amitryptyline

55. Which musculoskeletal disorder is considered an "auto-immune" disorder?
    a. Rheumatoid arthritis
    b. spondyloarthropathies
    c. tendontitis
    d. osteoarthritis

56. Determine the BSA for a child whose weight is 36 lb and height is 26 inches.
    a. 0.81 m^2
    b. 0.55 m^2
    c. 0.51 m^2
    d. 0.50 m^2

57. Fluticasone, triamcinolone and budesonide are classified as:
    a. anticholinergic
    b. leukotriene inhibitors
    c. anti-inflammatory
    d. antiallergic agents

58. 45 mL is equal to ___ L
    a. 45,000 L
    b. 450 L
    c. 0.045 L
    d. 0.45 L

59. Dextrose is the base component of TPN solutions most commonly given as a source of carbohydrates. Which of the following statements is true?
    a. it is available as a 5% solution that is commonly used in TPN solutions
    b. it is available in a concentrated form (50% or more) that is diluted in the final TPN solution to approximately 25%
    c. it is available as a 70% solution that is commonly given as a separate infusion for calories and energy
    d. all of the above

60. The generic name for Ritalin is:
    a. pyrodistigmine
    b. methylphenidate
    c. edrophonium
    d. glatiramer

61. Labeling an IV admixture should contain all of the following information *except*:
    a. patient name
    b. name and amount of drug(s) added
    c. prescribing physician's name
    d. expiration date

62. Contact with cytotoxic drugs can cause:
    a. dermatitis
    b. dizziness
    c. nausea
    d. all of the above

63. Which drug is classified as an anti-epileptic?
    a. Clonazepam
    b. Depakote
    c. Serevent
    d. Singulair

64. How long are records maintained after the expiration date for drug product components?
    a. three months
    b. six months
    c. one year
    d. three years

65. Convert 35 degrees Fahrenheit to Celsius.
    a. 2° C
    b. 6° C

c. 4° C
d. 10° C

66. What drug class does Immodium fall into?
    a. serotonin agonist
    b. antidiarrheal
    c. antiemetic
    d. H-2 blocker
    e. anticholinergic

67. Small volume parenterals are called:
    a. Add-Vantage
    b. LVP
    c. piggyback system
    d. none of the above

68. The goal of PCA is to:
    a. relieve pain as soon as the patient recognizes a need for it
    b. prevent a nurse of giving a shot
    c. prevent medication errors are delivering a calculated dosage
    d. allow nurses to carry out other duties

69. The brand name for diazepam is:
    a. Valium
    b. Ultram
    c. Cytoxan
    d. Vioxx
    e. Arava

70. A ___ is a particular way of accomplishing something or acting; a series of steps followed in a regular definite order; a traditional or established way of doing things.
    a. policy
    b. procedure

71. A package insert is required to be given to all patients who are taking:
    a. steroids
    b. analgesics
    c. estrogenic drugs
    d. all of the above

72. The generic name for Norvasc is:
    a. cyclophosphamide
    b. clopidogrel
    c. leflunamide
    d. amiodipine

73. How many tablespoons are in 45 mL?
    a. 2
    b. 3
    c. 5
    d. 10

74. The responsibilities of the State Board of Pharmacy include:
    a. licensure and registration of pharmacies
    b. dealing with complaints of professional misconduct
    c. labeling
    d. all of the above

75. Which drug falls into the class of opiods?
    a. Darvocet N-100
    b. Deltasone
    c. Voltaren

d. Klonopin

e. Cuprimine

76. Calculate the completion time for the following infusion. An IV with a restart time of 9:07 p.m. has an infusion time of 6 hr 27 min.

a. 3:34 p.m.

b. 12:37 p.m.

c. 2:34 p.m.

d. 3:34 a.m.

77. Calculate the BSA for a child weighing 14.2 kg and whose height is 64 cm.

a. 0.49 m^2

b. 0.50 m^2

c. 0.55 m^2

d. 0.65 m^2

78. Drugs that end in "am" are classified as:

a. Tricyclic antidepressants

b. MAOI

c. Antidepressants

d. Benzodiazepines

79. What is the completion time for an IV that started at 1450 and has an infusion time of 3 hr 40 min?

a. 1530

b. 1830

c. 2000

d. 2150

80. The ___ only needs to be functionally separate from non-sterile product preparation and constructed to minimize particulate and microbial contamination.

a. clean room

b. sterile compounding area

81. Remeron, Celexan, and Serzone are all classified as:

a. antianxiety

b. antimanics

c. antipsychotics

d. antidepressants

82. The CADD is an example of what type of pump system?

a. mechanical system

b. electronic controlled pressure and chemical release system

c. ambulatory electronic infusion pump system

d. none of the above

83. The *most* common complication of tunneled venous access devices are:

a. catheter occlusion (clogging)

b. infections

c. dislodgement (moving out of the vein)

d. venous thrombosis (blood clots)

84. The generic name for Prozac is:

a. fluoxetine

b. nefazodone

c. budesonide

d. rizatriptan

85. Convert 90 mL to ounces.

a. 27 oz

b. 30 oz

c. 3 oz

d. 15 oz

86. Change 4:36 to a percentage.

a. 8%

b. 11.1%

c. 9%

d. 111%

87. The brand name for famciclovir is:

a. Epivir HB

b. Cytovene

c. Novir

d. Famvir

88. Change 5:15 to a percentage.

a. 33.3%

b. 39%

c. 3%

d. 3.3%

89. The space between the HEPA filter and the sterile product being prepared is referred to as the:

a. hot spot

b. backwash zone

c. zone of turbulence

d. critical area

90. What class of drugs are Fungizone, Grasactin, and Nizoral in?

a. antifungals

b. non-nucleoside reverse transcriptase inhibitors

c. protease inhibitors

d. antivirals

91. Electolytes are added to TPN solutions to meet metabolic needs and correct deficiencies. Examples include:

a. amino acids

b. potassium chloride

c. vitamin D

d. lipid emulsions

92. Lipid or fat emulsions are typically administered by all of the following methods *except*:

a. as a 10% emulsion given through a peripheral line

b. as a 20% emulsion given through a peripheral line

c. as part of a 3-in-1 solution

d. IV push

93. The brand name for terbinafine is:

a. Viramune

b. Videx

c. Lamisil

d. Invirase

94. 65 mg is = to ___ mcg

a. 0.065 mcg

b. 0.65 mcg

c. 6500 mcg

d. 65,000 mcg

95. Protective apparel for those preparing cytotoxic or hazardous injections in a BSC includes:

a. a low permeability, solid front gown with tight fitting elastic cuffs

b. latex gloves

c. a self-contained respirator

d. both a & b

96. The generic name for Diflucan is:
    a. amantadine
    b. fluconazole
    c. amphotericin B
    d. ketoconazole

97. The ___ packaging system contains one dose of the drug for a given patient.
    a. single-dose
    b. single-unit
    c. individual wrap
    d. none of the above

98. When determining the gauge of the needle:
    a. the larger the number, the larger the size.
    b. the larger the number, the smaller the size.
    c. the smaller the number, the smaller the size.
    d. the smaller the number, the larger the size.

99. What is the brand name for anamtadine?
    a. Diflucan
    b. Sporanox
    c. Fungizone
    d. Symmetrel

100. Preservatives in parenteral products:
    a. kill organisms and therefore eliminate the need for aseptic technique and LAHs
    b. are harmless and non-toxic in any amount
    c. are present in multi-dose vials
    d. all of the above are correct

101. Which of the following statements concerning narcotic control is true?
    a. A separate control system for CII drugs is not desirable.
    b. It is not necessary to restrict access to records.
    c. Automated dispensing systems are frequently used for narcotic control.
    d. Narcotics have the same refill guidelines non-scheduled drugs.

102. The generic name for Nolvadex is:
    a. tamoxifen
    b. mercaptopurine
    c. carboplatin
    d. cisplatin

103. The pharmacy is asked to prepare a dosage of 85 mg. The pharmacy stocks 0.1 g/1.5 mL. How many milliliters does the technician need to prepare?
    a. 1.2 mL
    b. 1.3 mL
    c. 1.4 mL
    d. 1.5 mL

104. The clinical section contains those activities involved in patient-related monitoring activities of a clinical nature. Examples include:
    a. drug information services
    b. drug ordering
    c. unit-dose drug distribution
    d. none of the above

105. The classification for Symmetrel is:
    a. antibiotic
    b. antifungal
    c. protease inhibitor
    d. antiviral

106. In hospitals that use large amounts of tax-free alcohol, which department is responsible for the dispensing and storage of the alcohol?
    a. dietary
    b. pharmacy
    c. administration
    d. lab

107. The Durham-Humphrey Amendments provides:
    a. additional safeguards for prescription and over-the-counter drugs.
    b. information regarding the storage and distribution of controlled substances
    c. requirements for child-resistant packaging
    d. guidelines for pharmacists on counseling for patients.

108. The brand name for atorvastatin is:
    a. Toprol XL
    b. Lipitor
    c. Lanoxin
    d. Plavix

109. The federal regulatory agency responsible for controlling tax-free alcohol is the:
    a. Bureau of Alcohol, Tobacco and Firearms (ATF)
    b. Food and Drug Administration (FDA)
    c. Joint Commission on Accreditation of Healthcare Organizations (JCAHO)
    d. Drug Enforcement Administration (DEA)

110. How many micrograms are in 50 milligrams?
    a. 50,000 mcg
    b. 500 mcg
    c. 0.050 mcg
    d. 5000 mcg

111. The brand name for clopidogrel is:
    a. Lipitor
    b. Toprol XL
    c. Plavix
    d. Lanoxin

112. For drugs to be given via an ambulatory infusion device, ___ hour stability at room temperature or warmer is required.
    a. 12 hr
    b. 24 hr
    c. 36 hr
    d. 48 hr

113. The primary or natural pacemaker of the heart is the:
    a. sinoatrial note (SA node)
    b. atrioventricular node (AV node)
    c. bundle branches
    d. purkinje fibers

114. Norvasc, Cardizem, and Adalat belong to which class of drugs?
    a. ACE inhibitors
    b. alpha blockers
    c. beta blockers
    d. calcium channel blockers

115. Large volume parenteral solution containers with potent drugs that need to be infused with a high degree of accuracy and precision are usually administered with the aid of a:
    a. roller clamp
    b. electronic infusion device
    c. these solutions are not given IV
    d. LAH

116. Parental drug products should be:
    a. free of particulate matter
    b. sterile
    c. free of pyrogens
    d. all of the above

117. Which drug is classified as a Loop Diuretic?
    a. guanadrel
    b. chlorthalidone
    c. furosemide
    d. timolol

118. Before working in the LAH:
    a. interior surfaces should be wiped with 70% isopropyl alcohol
    b. the hood should be operated for at least 15-30 minutes
    c. hands should be washed in bactericidal soap
    d. all of the above

119. Items inside a LAH should be placed away from other objects and the walls of the hood to prevent:
    a. zone of turbulence
    b. dead space
    c. window of contamination
    d. laminar air

120. Which drug listed below is classified as an ACE inhibitor?
    a. Coreg
    b. Midamore
    c. Mavik
    d. Quinaglute

121. Mixing of 3-in-1 solutions should be performed carefully to prevent the emulsion "oiling out". It is recommended that this be accomplished by:
    a. preparing the solution in a very cold room
    b. preparing the solution from fresh lipids
    c. using a mixing order of fats, amino acids, and then dextrose
    d. using a mixing order of dextrose, fats, and then amino acids

122. Chest pain due to insufficient blood flow in the coronary arteries that is reversible with the administration of nitroglycerin is called:
    a. Angina Pectoris
    b. Myocardial infarction
    c. Arteriosclerosis
    d. Congestive Heart Failure

123. Which drug listed below is classified as a thiazide diuretic?
    a. chlorthalidone
    b. timolol
    c. guanadrel
    d. nicardipine

124. Convert 32 degrees Fahrenheit to Celsius.
    a. 2° C
    b. 0° C
    c. -4° C
    d. 6° C

125. After a cytotoxic agent is prepared in the pharmacy, transportation:
    a. should be done immediately
    b. should be done in a way as to minimize breakage
    c. includes making the transporter aware of what they are carrying and what the procedure would be in the event of a spill
    d. both b & c

Practice Exam Answer Key

1. a	48. c	95. d
2. a	49. a	96. b
3. c	50. b	97. a
4. b	51. d	98. b
5. b	52. c	99. d
6. a	53. a	100. c
7. a	54. b	101. c
8. d	55. a	102. a
9. c	56. b	103. b
10. d	57. c	104. a
11. a	58. c	105. d
12. b	59. b	106. b
13. c	60. b	107. a
14. b	61. c	108. b
15. d	62. d	109. a
16. b	63. b	110. a
17. b	64. c	111. c
18. c	65. a	112. b
19. b	66. b	113. a
20. a	67. c	114. d
21. c	68. a	115. b
22. d	69. a	116. d
23. c	70. b	117. c
24. d	71. c	118. d
25. a	72. d	119. a
26. a	73. b	120. c
27. b	74. d	121. c
28. c	75. a	122. a
29. a	76. d	123. a
30. d	77. b	124. b
31. b	78. d	125. d
32. d	79. b	
33. a	80. b	
34. b	81. d	
35. a	82. c	
36. d	83. b	
37. a	84. a	
38. c	85. c	
39. b	86. b	
40. a	87. d	
41. a	88. a	
42. d	89. d	
43. b	90. a	
44. c	91. b	
45. b	92. d	
46. c	93. c	
47. a	94. d	

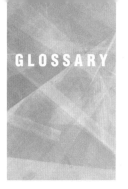

A

additive drug reaction – when the combined effect of two drugs is equal to the sum of the separate effects of the two drugs

adverse effect – any undesirable effect of a drug

afferent neurons – neurons that relay information to the CNS

Alzheimer disease – progressive neurological disorder that results from the degeneration of the cerebral cortex and hippocampus and low levels of the neurotransmitter acetycholine

anatomy – the study of body structure

antagonistic drug reaction – when one drug interferes with another, causing the effects of one of the drugs to be lessened or completely neutralized

apothecaries' system – used before the metric system was introduced; used to measure liquid volume (unit is the minim) and solid weight (unit is the grain)

area of turbulence – a triangular–shaped area in front of the beaker in which is a mixture of HEPA air and unfiltered room air

aseptic technique – a method used to prevent the contamination of an object by microorganisms

asthma – an inflammatory disorder that affects the bronchial tubes of the lungs, characterized by bronchospasms, airway constriction, mucous membrane swelling, and increased mucus production

automated dispensing systems – storage, dispensing, and charging devices for medications

autonomic nervous system (ANS) – responsible for involuntary control of smooth muscle, cardiac muscle, and glands

avoirdupois system – means goods sold by weight, used for ordering and purchasing some pharmaceutical products and for weighing patients

B

bar codes – unique arrangements of lines used to identify the item on which they are printed

biological safety cabinet (BSC) – a type of hood that blows HEPA-filtered air vertically downward through a top hood and into grills located along the front and back edges of the work surface area and that has a clear glass or plastic shield

biometric access – authentication technique that relies on measurable physical characteristics (such as a fingerprint) that can be automatically checked

body substance isolation – the practice of isolating all body substances (blood, urine, feces, tears, etc.) of individuals who might be infected with illnesses to reduce the chances of transmitting these illnesses

body surface area (BSA) – the area covered by a person's external skin

bradycardia – a heart rate of less than 60 beats per minute

brand name – the name a manufacturer assigns to a drug

buccal – drug administration in the pouch between the cheek and the gum

C

capitation – the annual fee paid to a physician or group of physicians by each participant in a health plan

capsule – a pill-like shell that contains a liquid or powder form of medication; dissolves when it reaches the stomach, releasing the medication

catheter – a delivery or drainage tube that is inserted into a vein, artery, or body cavity

central nervous system (CNS) – the brain and spinal chord

Certified Pharmacy Technicians (CPhT) – credential given to pharmacy technicians who have passed the Pharmacy Technician Certification Exam (PTCE); initial certification and recertification last for two years

civil laws – laws that govern wrongdoings against a person or property, and generally charges are brought forth by another individual

Class A prescription balance scale – scale required by law for use in the pharmacy to weigh out dosages of solid medications

clean room – an area in which the air quality, temperature, and humidity are highly regulated to reduce the risk of cross-contamination

community pharmacists – stand-alone businesses that fill prescriptions as well as nonprescription products for ambulatory patients

compound sterile product (CSP) – a mixture of one or more substances that is made sterile, or free of contamination, before use

congestive heart failure (CHF) – condition that results from the heart's inability to pump enough blood to vital parts of the body, often leading to an increase in blood pressure and an excess retention of fluid in the lungs, liver, and other parts of the body

contaminant – any unwanted particulate matter or sickness-inducing agent

continuous quality improvement – a scientific and systematic process of monitoring, evaluating, and identifying problems and then developing and measuring the impact of the improvement strategies

contraindications – reasons for not giving a particular drug to a patient, such as allergic reactions or preexisting conditions

controlled-release medications – drugs designed to release at a constant, gradual rate over an extended period of time

Controlled Substances Act (CSA) – 1970 act that was designed to help regulate drug use by creating rules and regulations for record keeping and dispensing, and requiring firms that handled controlled substances to register with the DEA; the act also organized controlled substances into a system of schedules based on the potential for abuse

coronary artery disease (CAD) – condition affecting the blood vessels that feed the heart muscle, allowing a build-up of plaque inside the vessels that over time causes them to narrow, thicken, and become unable to carry blood to other parts of the body

crash carts – trays used by all areas of a hospital that contain injectable medications used for a code blue (respiratory distress)

critical area – a place where CSPs, containers, and closures are exposed to the environment

critical site – location where contaminants might come into contact with a CSP

D

diabetes – a disorder of the pancreas involving production of insulin

dimensional analysis – method of problem solving used when two quantities are directly proportional to each other

disease – anything that upsets the structure or function of a part, organ, or system of the body

disinfection – the use of liquid chemicals on surfaces and at room temperature to kill disease-causing microorganisms

drip rate – the number of drops of solution infused per minute

Drug Enforcement Administration (DEA) – agency of the United States government that controls who may prescribe, distribute, and fill prescriptions for controlled or scheduled drugs in the United States

drug indications – reasons for giving a particular drug to a patient

Drug Listing Act – 1972 act established to create a list of marketed drugs for the Food and Drug Administration, which would assist with enforcing federal safety laws

Durham-Humphrey Amendment (DHA) – 1951 amendment that separated drugs into two categories: legend drugs (prescriptions drugs) and over-the-counter drugs (OTC); the amendment specified that news drugs can only be distributed through prescriptions (and should contain legends to that effect), but eventually may be changed to OTC status

E

efferent neurons – neurons that carry information from the CNS to muscles and glands

elixir – drug dissolved in alcohol and flavored

emphysema – a chronic obstructive pulmonary disorder that occurs when the alveoli are permanently enlarged due to exposure to outside irritants like cigarette smoke or air pollution

emulsion – medication that is combined with water and oil

enteral medications – drugs that enter the body through the gastrointestinal tract

epidemiology – the study of epidemics caused by infectious agents, toxic agents, air pollution, and other health-related phenomena

ergodynamics – the applied science concerned with designing and arranging equipment and people so that they can work efficiently and safely

ethics – system of values, principles, and duties that guide behavior

explosive substances – release sudden pressure, gaseous elements, and heat when subjected to shock, hot or high pressure

extract – a highly concentrated form of a medication, typically given in a liquid to hide its strong taste

F

fee-for-service – an insurance plan in which the patient pays out of pocket for services and then submits for reimbursement separately from the insurance plan

flammable and combustible substances – those that are easy to ignite, for example paint thinners, charcoal, lighter fluid, and silver polish

flexible spending account – a pretax-funded account that allows an employee to set aside a portion of his or her earnings to pay for qualified medical expenses

flow rate – the number of milliliters of fluids administered per hour or per minute

Food, Drug, and Cosmetic Act (FDCA) – 1938 act that helped ensure drugs being distributed were safe and fulfilled the reported claim of strength, purity, and quality

Food and Drug Administration (FDA) – agency of the United States government that controls the drugs that are acceptable for use in the United States; the two criteria the administration assures are the safety and efficiency of a drug

formulary – a list of approved drug products stocked by a pharmacy

G

gastroesophageal reflux disease (GERD) – a condition in which the gastric contents of the stomach, including acid, back up or reflux into the esophagus

generic name – the official name assigned to a drug

H

hazardous material – any substance or mixture of substances having properties capable of producing adverse effects on the health and safety or the environment of a human being

high-efficiency particulate air (HEPA) filter – a special filter that traps all particles larger than 0.2 μm

Health Insurance Portability and Accountability Act (HIPAA) – act established in 1996 that requires healthcare providers to provide a clear written explanation of how health information will be used and disclosed

HEPA – filtered high-efficiency particulate air

home health pharmacy – pharmacies that are based away from hospital sites and not open to the public, couriers deliver the medications to the home health clients

hypothyroidism – a condition in which there is a deficiency of thyroid hormone

hyperthyroidism – a condition in which there is an increase in the amount of thyroid hormones manufactured and secreted

I

inert ingredients – also called pharmaceutical ingredients, non-medicinal agents delivered in combination with drug substances, e.g., preservatives

infection control – factors related to the spread of infections within the healthcare setting

infectious waste – includes blood, blood products and body fluids, infectious sharps waste, laboratory waste, and animal waste

infusion pump – an automatic device used with an IV system for delivering medication at regular intervals in specific quantities

infusion time – volume to be infused divided by flow rate

inpatient pharmacy – pharmacy located in a hospital where patients stay overnight or longer; have a wider range of stock than outpatient pharmacies because they provide the specific medication and supplies for every department in the hospital

intramuscular (IM) – drug administration by injection into muscle

intravenous (IV) – drug administration directly into the blood through a vein

intravenous push (IVP) – a small volume of medicine injected into a vein and administered over a short period of time

intravenous piggybacks (IVPB) – administered on a set schedule, smaller IV bags that are added on, or "piggybacked," to a large-volume IV bag

inventory – the quantity and type of substances on hand in the pharmacy

investigational drugs – drugs that have not yet been approved by the FDA for human use

investigational product – a pharmaceutical form of an active ingredient or placebo tested and used as a reference in a clinical trial

K

Kefauver-Harris Amendment (KHA) – 1962 amendment that became part of the Food, Drug, and Cosmetic Act; the amendment was designed to institute higher safety measures for drugs approved by the Food and Drug Administration by requiring manufacturers to follow Good Manufacturing Processes (GMP)

L

laminar airflow hood (LAH) – a work area that prefilters large contaminants from the workspace and then uses HEPA-filtered air in a horizontal flow to extract smaller particles

large-volume IV bag – often used for fluid replacement or for maintenance of fluids, administered continually

legend – a drug that can be dispensed to the public only with an order given by a properly authorized person

levigation – process to reduce particle size and grittiness of added powders for small scale preparation of ointments

M

mail-order pharmacy – large distribution pharmacies that dispense medication through the mail

managed care pharmacy – operate much like a community or other ambulatory care pharmacies, but carry only drugs that are on the organization's formulary and serve only patients covered on their plan

manufacturer recalls – occur when there is a problem in the manufacture or distribution of a drug product that may present a risk to public health

Material Safety Data Sheets (MSDS) – forms containing data regarding the properties of particular substances

master gland – the pituitary gland, which releases the hormones that affect how other glands work

mechanism of action – the way a drug works

medical orders – the means of communication between the pharmacy and physicians in an institutional setting whereby medical procedures and prescription medications are described

metric system – most widely used system for measuring drugs, a decimal system based on the number 10 and multiples and subdivisions of 10

multidose packaging system – drug packaging system in which medication is distributed in single-dose packing but where the dose is more than one unit

multiple-dose vials – vials that allow access to the contents of the vial more than once

N

National Drug Code (NDC) – the unique numerical code assigned by manufacturers to each drug they produce

non-unit-dose distribution system – drug packaging system in which medication is distributed in bulk bottles

O

Occupational Safety and Health Administration (OSHA) – government agency within the United States Department of Labor responsible for maintaining safe and healthy work environments

Orphan Drug Act – 1983 act created by the Food and Drug Administration to speed up the approval process for new medications intended to help people with urgent needs

osteoporosis – a bone disorder in which bones become fragile due to a lack of normal calcium salt deposits and a decrease in bone protein

outpatient pharmacy – a pharmacy that is not connected with a hospital

over-the-counter (OTC) medications – medications that do not require a prescription to be purchased

P

paraprofessional – a person who is trained to assist professionals but is not licensed at a professional level

parasympathetic nervous system – part of the autonomic nervous system (ANS), includes fibers that originate in the brain stem and sacral regions of the spinal cord

parenteral medications – drugs that do not pass through the gastrointestinal tract, e.g., injections, inhalants, and topical creams

par levels – predetermined quantities of medications that should be kept in stock

Parkinson disease – progressive neurologic disorder usually caused by the death of cells in the part of the brain that produces dopamine

percent – parts per hundred; another way to express fractions and numerical relationships

periodic automatic replenishment level – the minimum amount of medication that a pharmacy should have in stock at any given time

peripheral nervous system (PNS) – all nerves other than the brain and spinal chord

perpetual inventory – a method to manage the stock of controlled substances on a continuous basis wherein each time a controlled substance is received or dispensed, it is recorded in a computerized system

personal protective equipment (PPE) – specialized clothing or equipment worn by healthcare workers for protection against a hazard by creating a physical barrier

pharmaceutic phase – with non-liquid oral medications, the body's dissolution of the drug so that the body can absorb it

pharmaceutical business – merges the fields of health care and business, combining the key elements of pharmaceutical-science and pharmaceutical-marketing programs

pharmaceutical companies – specialize in the research, development, and marketing of medicines

pharmaceutical equivalent – medications that have identical active ingredients, dosages, and routes of administration

pharmaceuticals manufacturers – take raw materials and process them into finished medicines ready for the consumer

pharmacodynamic phase – the drug's effects on the body

pharmacokinetic phase – the process of how the body handles the drug, includes absorption, distribution, metabolism, and excretion

pharmacology – the study of drugs and how they work in therapeutic use

pharmacy satellite – a designated area with patient care where drugs are stored, prepared, and dispensed for patients

Pharmacy Technician Certification Board (PTCB) – governing body that was formed in 1995 to establish national standards for pharmacy technician certification

Pharmacy Technician Certification Exam (PTCE) – certification exam designed to test the skills required for pharmacy technicians; after passing the exam, a pharmacy technician is certified by the Pharmacy Technician Certification Board (PTCB)

poisons – also known as or toxic materials, can cause injury or death when they enter the bodies of living things

physiology – the study of how the body functions

Poison Prevention Packaging Act (PPPA) – 1970 act created to reduce potential for accidental poisonings

policy – a high-level, overall plan, and a definite course or method of action selected from among alternatives

policies and procedures (P&P) – documents provided by an institution to give guidance to personnel regarding what is expected of them

potentiation – the process of one drug becoming more effective through the simultaneous administration of another drug

procedure – a traditional or standard way of doing things

Q

quality control – the process of checks and balances followed during the manufacturing of a product or the delivery of a service to ensure that the end product or services meets or exceeds previously determined standards

quality improvement – a scientific and systematic process involving monitoring, evaluating, and identifying problems and then developing and measuring the improvement strategies

R

radiopharmaceuticals – unique medicinal formulations containing radioisotopes used in major clinical areas for diagnosis and/or therapy

registration – the process of being enrolled in an existing list of accepted pharmacy technicians who have met the standards of a particular state

reorder point – the quantity at which a product should be reordered to maintain minimum acceptable quantity in the pharmacy

risk level – the potential risk to patients caused by the introduction of microbial contamination into a finished sterile product

S

Schedule of Controlled Substances – a five-category listing of drugs according to their potential for abuse and usage in the United States

single-dose vials – contain one dose of medication and are discarded after one use

solid waste – a term used by the U.S. Environmental Protection Agency (EPA) to define all solid, liquid, and gaseous waste

solubility – the property of a substance that can be dissolved in a liquid to form a homogenous solution

solution – a liquid form of medication that contains medications in a water base

somatic nervous system – responsible for voluntarily control of the skeletal system

standard precautions – are the minimum required level of infection control in all settings and all situations, and thus define safe work practices regardless of known or presumed infectious status

sterile – free from contaminants

sterilization – a process intended to kill all microorganisms and is the highest level of microbial kill that is possible

stroke – brain disorder, also called a cerebrovascular accident, usually caused by a blockage of blood flow to certain areas of brain tissue

subcutaneous (SubQ or SC) – drug administration by injection beneath the skin into subcutaneous tissue, usually in the patient's upper arm, thigh, or abdomen

sublingual (SL) – drug administration under the tongue

suspensions – drugs that have been finely divided and placed in a liquid or fluid vehicle; oral suspensions are usually water-based, but suspensions intended for other purposes can have different vehicles

sympathetic nervous system – part of the ANS, includes fibers that originate in the thoracic and lumbar regions of the spinal cord

synergistic drug reaction – when the combined effect of two drugs is greater than the sum of the separate effects of the two drugs

syrup – sweet, flavored forms of liquid medication

T

tablets – form of medication that is a solid, such as a pill

tachycardia – a heart rate of more than 100 beats per minute

therapeutic effect – the intended effect in the treatment of a symptom or illness

third-party billing – billing a patient's insurance company for products and services

third-party programs – insurance or entitlement programs that reimburse the pharmacy for products delivered and services rendered

tincture – a total alcohol solution

topical – drug administration through the skin of mucous membrane

total nutrition admixture (TNA) – also known as total parenteral nutrition, IV therapy that provides nutrition to patients who cannot take nourishment by mouth

total parenteral nutrition (TPN) – also known as total nutrition admixture, IV therapy that provides nutrition to patients who cannot take nourishment by mouth

transdermal – drug administration of ointment, cream, or gel through the skin using a patch that releases the drug gradually

twenty-four-hour time – also called military time, method of keeping time by numbering the hours from 1 to 24 rather than 1 to 12 twice

U

unit-dose system – a packaging system in which medication is dispensed in a single dose package that is ready to administer to the patient

United States Pharmacopeia (USP) – non-governmental, official public standard-setting authority for prescription and over-the-counter medicines and other healthcare products manufactured or sold in the United States